The Biodynamic Philosophy
and Treatment of

Biodynamic Psychology and Psychotherapy

edited by

Mary Molloy
Institute of Biodynamic
Psychology and Psychotherapy

Volume 1

PETER LANG
Bern · Berlin · Bruxelles · Frankfurt am Main · New York · Oxford · Wien

Peg Nunneley

The Biodynamic Philosophy and Treatment of Psychosomatic Conditions

Volume 1

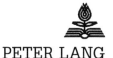

PETER LANG

Bern · Berlin · Bruxelles · Frankfurt am Main · New York · Oxford · Wien

Die Deutsche Bibliothek – CIP-Einheitsaufnahme

Nunneley, Peg:
The biodynamic philosophy and treatment of psychosomatic conditions
/ Peg Nunneley. – Bern ; Berlin ; Bruxelles ; Frankfurt am Main ; New
York ; Oxford ; Wien : Lang, 2000
(Biodynamic psychology and psychotherapy ; Vol. 1)
ISBN 3-906763-16-1

British Library and Library of Congress Cataloguing-in-Publication
Data: A catalogue record for this book is available from *The British
Library*, Great Britain, and from *The Library of Congress*, USA

ISSN 1424-6279
ISBN 3-906763-16-1
US-ISBN 0-8204-4608-4

© Peter Lang AG, European Academic Publishers, Bern 2000
Jupiterstr. 15, Postfach, 3000 Bern 15, Switzerland; info@peterlang.com

Printed in Germany

Foreword to the Book Series – Biodynamic Psychology and Psychotherapy

Biodynamic Psychology and Psychotherapy presents a psychological and somatic approach to the health of the human organism in its environment. It is based on the theories and insights of the founder of the biodynamic concepts and practices, Gerda Boyesen.

Mrs Boyesen is a Norwegian Clinical Psychologist, Reichian Analyst and Physiotherapist. For the past 40 years she has developed her unique concepts and techniques.

Originally based upon the theories of Freud, Jung and Reich the essential contribution of the Gerda Boyesen insights is the concept of a physical manifestation of the unconscious, the *'Id'*. Freud and Reich looked for this manifestation but did not find it.

The first two books in this Series have been written by Peg Nunneley. Mrs Nunneley's writings demonstrate the somatic and psychological techniques that can he used when treating some psychosomatic conditions.

Further books in the series will include a second volume of selected writings by Peg Nunneley followed by other authors. There will be a series of manuals and textbooks, post-graduate dissertations, writings about specialist and related topics and the launch of a new Journal, the 'Journal of Biodynamic Psychotherapy'.

Mary Molloy
Series Editor
London 2000

*In ancient times
the thunderbolt was the symbol of Illumination.*

Hellenic Mithraism

Acknowledgements

To my parents who nourished us and especially my father who taught us to have curiosity.

He once woke the whole family to see the Aurora Borealis hovering beyond the coastline of North Wales.

Contents

Confidentiality

In the interests of protecting the privacy and confidentiality of patients, names and identifying details have been eliminated or disguised.

Introduction: the Biodynamic approach

Bio ... means Life
Dynamic ... Movement

Biodynamic means the spontaneous, natural flow of life energy, life force or bio-energy through the body, mind, spirit, soul and organism.
In 1872 Herbert Spencer [1] wrote:

> A living thing is distinguished from a dead thing by the multiplicity of the changes at any one moment taking place in it.

The term biodynamic describes a living process of natural health and well being. When the harmonious flow of this life energy is disturbed, the organism may experience pain on the physical, mental and spiritual levels.

Gerda Boyesen, the founder of Biodynamic Psychology, introduced the term 'psycho-peristalsis' to describe an actual healing mechanism in the core of the body, in the alimentary tract. The biodynamic practitioner uses a stethoscope placed over the lower abdomen to monitor sounds from the gut as a therapeutic technique is used.

Gerda Boyesen realised that the alimentary tract not only digests nutrients, but is also the conduit for the unconscious, the 'id'. This secondary function has the capacity to digest the hormonal remnants and by-products of emotional stress. It is a vital factor in maintaining the body's ability to balance and harmonise the organism even after the most severe emotional and physical trauma. Health means the ability to express, resolve and digest.

These chapters describe some of the therapeutic tools with which the biodynamic practitioner interprets and treats dysfunctions in the human organism.

Training takes place over a five-year period. Students are committed to their own personal therapeutic involvement, as well as to becoming proficient in the skills of the work. A five-year programme of learn-

---

1   Spencer, Herbert, *Principles of Biology,* London, 1872.

ing the physiotherapeutic and psychotherapeutic techniques maintain the high standard of Gerda Boyesen's conceptual brilliance.

Preface

This is a collection of writings recorded over the years and which attempts to describe the way that Biodynamic Psychology and Psychotherapy come together in the treatment of psychosomatic conditions. It is important to recognise that the title of these first two books in the series does not encompass the range of psychotherapeutic intentions and techniques for which we are trained.

There are many ways of treating illnesses. I write from the life experience of being a nurse and nursing sister, with a specialist training in orthopaedic nursing, and as a psychologist with psychoanalytic training.

In 1973 I met Gerda Boyesen and subsequently trained with her at the *Gerda Boyesen Centre* in London. When Gerda Boyesen's insights into the workings of the body, mind and soul-spirit came into my life, many of the hitherto inexplicable illnesses – sometimes known as idiopathic conditions, became less mysterious, less inexplicable. Mysteries remained, but a logic – a biologic – seemed to run through the person's breakdown into illness and away from wellness and wellbeing.

It seemed that health was no longer to be seen as an absence of illness, but rather as an ability to progress through the illness, using it to move forward and beyond whatever it was that had caused a breakdown of communication between systems and cells.

This collection of papers also comes from the experience of balancing an orthodox view of some illnesses with new philosophers, such as Rupert Sheldrake and the late David Bohm and their cosmic perceptions.

Gerda Boyesen recognised the physical manifestation of the unconscious (the id) when she posited that the gut was the canal for the id energies. Conflicts arise and can lead to disease when the central nervous system, the ego, is out of synchrony with the id. The humanness of the conscience, the superego, can cause disturbance and dysfunction in the huge intelligence of cell communication.

Biodynamic psychologists and psychotherapists are brought face to face with the results of this disturbance in their every day experiences with sick and unhappy people. A deep chasm continues to inhibit communication between much of orthodox medicine and a complementary approach to human ills, such as that practised by biodynamic psychology and psychotherapy. There is growing evidence that scientific studies are beginning to validate some of the Gerda Boyesen concepts. The problem is that many centres of scientific studies have no knowledge of biodynamic concepts.

Communication is not happening – at least *almost* never. The 'almost' may be significant. It means that there is a door ajar. The emerging generation of physicians and surgeons are questioning old dogmas. The millennium may be the signal for communication.

Gerda Boyesen was born in Bergen in Norway on the eighteenth of May 1922. She graduated from *Oslo University* as a Clinical Psychologist and at the same time underwent a psychoanalytic training with Norway's eminent psychologist, Ola Raknes. Later, she trained as a physiotherapist at the *Oslo Orthopaedic Institute*.

In 1956 she studied some particularly significant new techniques at the *Bulow Hansen Institute* in Oslo. In the years following her training and clinical experiences in various hospitals and clinics, Gerda Boyesen developed her concepts and powerful new methods of treatment.

The purity and simplicity of her work has been maintained in the training of students of the *Institute of Biodynamic Psychology and Psychotherapy* in London and Killala in the west of Ireland.

Peg Nunneley
January 2000

Sit down before fact like a little child and be prepared to give up every precon-
ceived notion, follow humbly wherever and to whatever abyss nature leads or you
shall learn nothing.

T.H. Huxley

In the new view of health, we cease to see disease as entirely negative. Health, too,
is not altogether positive for us. The fact is that the distinctions between health and
disease at a point begin to blur. Why? For one reason we have come to see the im-
possibility of events such as health and disease as being local; that is; they are connected and dependent on all distant happenings in the universe.

This degree of connectedness suggests that good or bad health or disease are capri-
cious and arbitrary judgements. In the new view we attach little value to health and
disease rather than seeing them as either good or bad, to us they seem to be simply
a statement of the way things are.

For us this is not a statement of passivity and blind acceptance for we can still act
to change the physical state of the body. It is merely a feeling born of the recognition of the interpenetrating oneness of all things.

Larry Dossey, M.D., Space, Time and Medicine, 1982

CHAPTER 1

Or would you rather be a cat?

Once upon a time I had a cat called Thai Phu. She was a beautiful Siamese with an impeccable lineage. She came to see me together with some of her brothers and sisters. The lady breeder of this family had heard that I was looking for a Siamese kitten and had offered to bring the litter. The kittens were eight weeks old and nearly ready for adoption. I had never had a cat of my own though my country childhood had always included a variety of standoffish, variegated farm cats. In case my sitting room carpet could be a target in a kitten accident, I put down a tray of a mixture of paper and bulb fibre on the floor near my sitting room door and waited for my guests to arrive.

The lady breeder came in carrying a big cat basket containing four entrancing, leggy, little, coffee-coloured kittens. I soon realised that I was completely out of my depth here. I had no idea how it would be possible to choose one of these bundles of delicious energy and if I knew little about cats in general I knew nothing at all about this exotic variety. The mutual interview finally came to an end and I had been adopted with no say in the choosing. As the kittens were being gathered up from around the carpet, one of them went to the tray of paper and bulb fibre and pee-ed. Decision time...and I had been adopted. She arrived three days later.

From then on she followed me everywhere even to the post box round the corner, always at my heels. She became my familiar. Her kennel name was a bit over the top so finding a real name was an urgent matter. We were watching television the evening of her arrival and an advertisement for tea bags came up on the screen. We adapted it to Thai Phu. This tripped off the tongue very nicely and when I learned a little time later that a translation from the Thai was a bit rude, it was too late to change. Her wildness was evident in her instinctive behaviour but she compromised with my human-ness; and to the end she was my friend. She deserves a book all to herself.

My understanding of wildness in a cat prompts the writing of this article. What does this story of a kitten have to do with biodynamic psychology and psychotherapy? Gerda Boyesen, the Norwegian Clinical Psychologist, developed the philosophy and practice of biodynamic psychology and psychotherapy. One of the topics of Gerda Boyesen's research was on how life energy manifests itself? Here we are at the end and the beginning of a millennium of enormously important events in the history of mankind and the planet on which we live and we are still arguing about what it is that makes us alive.

This phenomenon called life is still not understood, and for the student of biodynamic psychology and philosophy it is difficult. The use of the words 'life energy' can limit any flow of dialogue that arises with scientists or anybody of orthodox philosophy. It is often a question of how each person in a dialogue perceives him or her self or the subject under scrutiny. Perception depends on the needs of the individual who perceives. If I complain that my garden is suffering from too much rainfall, I see the weather as my enemy. If I live in a drought area in Australia and my garden is dying, a week of heavy rainfall is heaven on earth. It is this difficulty that is inherent in conversations between biodynamic theorists and scientists which causes conversations to dry up. The protagonists are looking in opposite directions and curiosity about each other's point of view dies.

What, you may ask, does this have to do with Siamese cats, biodynamic psychology and life? Bear with me. I was once asked to go to see a neuro-physiologist in her university department. She had heard that I was convening an introductory workshop on biodynamic philosophy and its working practices. She and I met in her university laboratory. She said

I hear you are working with bio-plasma. How do you explain this?

In reply I said something like

I think this term is mostly in use in Russia. We use the term bio-energy or bio-dynamic but it all refers to life energy.

and I realised that I had dug myself a very big hole into which I was about to topple. Her next question was

And how do you describe this life energy?

Out of the corner of my right eye I saw some microscopes lying on a laboratory bench. I said

Imagine that you have two slides. One slide has some live cells in a medium. The other slide has dead cells in a medium. Under the lens of a microscope the live cells are enormously active. The dead cells show no such activity. The difference between the two slides is life.

I had some hope (or dread) that some kind of conversation would develop because I was out of my depth amongst all this paraphernalia. Instead I was stunned to hear her say

Can I offer you coffee in the cafeteria?

That was the sum total of our talk on life.

So, when writing this article, which attempts to describe life events through the activity of life energy I will do my utmost to keep the language simple. Especially where there are any physiological mechanisms not described in medical textbooks.

Life energy or 'prana' are terms familiar to yoga practitioners, and those who seek out the ancient medicine of China are familiar with the concept of the universal cosmic concept of 'chi' or 'ki'. It is a universal energy. The sciences of astronomy and astro-physics do not agree·about the fate of the cosmos but they currently agree that something energetic is happening, even in the countless areas in space, which were once seen as vacuums. Biodynamic psychology and psychotherapy is based on hypotheses conceived and developed by Gerda Boyesen. One basic tenet of biodynamic psychology and psychotherapy is that in attempting to understand and treat the neurotic patient, it is necessary to understand how malfunctions in the vegetative or autonomic nervous system have been the root cause of the illness and lack of wellbeing. More than this, it is necessary to understand that conflict between the nervous systems in the body is an inevitable result of being a human being. All living creatures have nervous systems and all living creatures have made some kind of adaptation to suit the species to which they belong.

One of these systems in our human organism is the vegetative or autonomic nervous system. It has developed so that we could be warned of imminent danger and the need to protect ourselves. We need a fast action mechanism if we are to survive. This is the primary function of the vegetative nervous system and it behaves in a particular manner. It has a four beat formula as follows:

stimulus – charge – discharge – recuperation

The primary emotion that stimulates a vegetative response is fear. It is the primal fear of possible extinction but is felt as an emotion and is a profound experience. To be able to perceive danger is a function of the other nervous system the central nervous system. We have a brain, a spinal cord and a peripheral nervous system. The latter picks up information from our body boundary with the outside world. This boundary is our skin, the largest organ in the body.

The two nervous systems develop more or less together in our embryological journey from conception onwards. The two systems work together for the common purpose of the survival of the individual and the species. The vegetative nervous system, composed of two parts, the sympathetic and the para-sympathetic, functions through specialised tracts of tissue and produces their individual hormones. The vegetative system governs such basic life functions as the heartbeat and to some extent, the taking in of oxygen through the lung function even when the central nervous system has ceased its function of communication. A patient is then said to be in a vegetative state.

All living creatures have these two systems, albeit in modified forms. From a meta-physical point of view we have developed philogenetically and ontologically through the aeons of life on this planet. The nervous systems were needed to explore and exploit the environment and then to adapt to whatever experiences were there, with the ultimate aim of survival. The development of these two systems was more or less simultaneous but although the intended functions are inter-dependent they are not identical. The phenomenon of fear is an experience felt as a result of the actions of the two nervous systems. It is an 'e-motion', a movement away from conflict. We do not feel a perception, we feel the results of what the central nervous system tells us. The vegetative system provides us with the opportunity to feel an emotion. As a result we may feel sad or glad or nothing. All of this is physiological. All living creatures need nervous systems in one modified form or another.

But...and here we come to the cat, at last! We humans are different from other creatures. The behaviour of a cat, particularly a wild cat, may illustrate the difference. Although my Siamese cat was wild and taught me a lot of things, she compromised in return for a more stable existence in a household of humans. Her compromises were limited, however. The cat of this story has compromised even less.

This is the story of a wild cat. This cat lives in the wild. We find it lying along a branch of a tree. Its muscles are relaxed as it sleeps in the warm sunshine. Suddenly, it jerks. It is awake. It has heard a sound from the ground below. It looks towards the place from which the sound has come. It sees a little movement. This is the function of its central nervous system. The cat has heard and seen. The perceptions have alerted the vegetative nervous system to respond. Wild animals have a constant need to find food. Nature is not always a reliable provider of food. The wild animal's search for food is endless and relentless. The cat's ears and eyes have stimulated and brought attention to the instinctive drive toward survival. For this cat the sounds and sights mean food.

Recalling the pattern of the four-beat formula this is the stimulus beat. This is the moment of stimulus. Action within the vegetative nervous system is instantaneous. This is the cat's instinctive response to the stimulus. Adrenalin is released into the bloodstream of the cat. This catalogue of events has been simplified in the telling. The release of adrenalin comes from the supra-renal glands, which sit on top of each kidney. There is no intermediate duct; the hormone goes straight into the bloodstream. The cat's muscular system has an immediate supply of the hormone and its sympathetic influence. The muscular system is primed and tensed and readied for action. This is the effect of one part of the vegetative nervous system and it is dramatic.

The cat is alert. Its stance is very attentive and very still. The power of the muscular system is contained. It holds its breath. Its heartbeat increases to send the hormone-charged blood into the muscle systems of the cat's body. It shuts down its digestive processes. Its blood pressure rises to maximise the flow of blood. Its fur stands on end and its whole body is tensed and poised very efficiently for action. This is the charge of the four-beat formula. The cat has no conflicting emotions. It jumps down on to the little animal that has moved and kills it. This is the completion of the charge and discharge of the four-beat formula.

Now, there is a reversal of the direction of the cat's instinctive responses. The up-going direction is reversed to a down-going one. The cat will digest the contents of its stomach...a downward direction. As human beings we can recall that we blush in an upward direction. This is a vegetative activity. The blushing disappears in a downward direction. The downward direction of the evidence of the flow is occasioned by the flow into the blood stream of another hormone. This comes from the action of another part of the vegetative nervous system. This is known as the parasympathetic nervous system. It produces a hormone called acetylcholine. The powerful adrenalin hormone has completed its task.

The antagonist acetylcholine is known to have a clearing effect and the adrenalin needs to be cleared from the cat's muscles in order that its efficient muscular mechanisms are assured. When this happens the discharge beat of the formula is complete. The cat is satisfied. Its stomach is full. Its instincts have been physically completed. It returns to the branch of the tree. It licks its chops and cleans itself. It is replete. It sleeps. Now is the time for recuperation. Recuperation. The fourth beat of the vegetative cycle. Until the next time.

I, however, am not a cat. I am a human being. I have all the primitive equipment of the two nervous systems at my disposal. I can see and hear. I am in reasonable working order and I can respond to danger with a release of the appropriate hormones. But...I do have a problem. I am a human being. My problem is that I have difficulty in completing the four-beat formula pattern or as it is also known, the startle reflex pattern. This is the situation. I have a comparatively, advanced and sophisticated development on many levels. I am in a tribe. This is different from the cat's pride or tribe. My developments in my tribe have produced advantages and disadvantages.

Because I am human, I have skills which enable me to communicate with other members of my tribe with a sophisticated form of language...and I am arrogant enough to think that the animal kingdom is not as clever as my tribe. I have tribal awareness, however, which the cat does not have, I have become careful of the members of my tribe. It is true that some animals are known to have caring skills. Elephants appear to have caring behaviour with sick and dying members of their families. They can be very territorial.

And now something has happened to me. I have a neighbour. He wants more territory for his family. He is a difficult chap to make friends with. He lives almost next door and he is trying to take over some of my land (stimulus)...and he is making me very angry (charge) so what do I do? What is the problem here? Well, now I have to suppress my instinctive animal response. I feel like killing him or running away from the aggravation that he is causing me...as far away as possible. It is at this point that human conflict arises. If I kill this man, his friends will come after me and, perhaps kill me. If I run away, my family will suffer and I have responsibilities.

The cat did not have this dialogue with himself. The difference, and perhaps the problem, is that I am a social animal. I have this thing called a conscience. I am a super-egoist person. I am dependent as a human being on having a super ego...a conscience. There are too many difficulties if I behave like the cat. If I make a fight or flee decision, the consequences will be too painful. So, I compromise. In so doing, I feel a little relief from the stress of having to make the big choice.

So, what will happen to the third stage of the four-beat formula? I have not cleared the biochemical remnants from my still tense muscles. What I actually do, very reluctantly, is let my neighbour take a piece of my land. He is happy. I tell myself that I have done the right thing. I have avoided blood shed or the long and painful flight. I have compromised and my conscience is clear...and I feel uneasy. Why? Well. I did not complete my instinctive instructions. In spite of my feeling that I have done the right thing the residue makes me feel uncomfortable. My intellect (my ego) has over-ridden my instincts and the result of making the compromise is the feeling of discomfort in my body and in my thinking processes, a little anxiety.

I could, perhaps, have removed some of the undischarged hormone remnants by shouting and screaming or having a very fast run. This would, at least, have increased my oxygen intake and loosened the tensions I feel in my chest. I could have had a good cry. This would have loosened the tensions in my facial tissues, which are still distorted by my angry facial expressions. There is the fluid factor to explain. What role do the tears play? I never saw Thai Phu cry. I continue to feel a little anxious and uncomfortable in my mind and in my body. It feels like unfinished business. I have not completed the discharge in the four-beat formula.

The result of this is an incomplete recuperation. This is where the seeds of neurosis are sown. This is the factor that is basic to the philosophy of biodynamic psychology. I do not learn my lesson from the experience with my neighbour. I continue to make the same compromising decisions over and over again. The miniscule remnants of the get up and go hormones are still hanging around. They eventually change biochemically and become an irritant. I now have pain and the feeling of mild anxiety. The pain eventually forces me to go and get some advice and help. I go to see the tribal doctor. He gives me advice and some medicine to help me get on with my work and caring for my family. I have disturbed the completion of the four-beat formula. In order to get back into the comfort zone I have moved into a fifth beat in the formula. I am now in rehabilitation.

Therapeutic intervention

My nervous systems struggle to maintain balance and harmony but I continue to behave unwisely. I take the medicine. I go to bed and sleep and hope to feel better in the morning. And for a while this works. I half trust nature to undo the damage caused by my unwise behaviour. I do know, vaguely, that the feelings of unease are of my own doing but my attention to this is easily distracted. Now I have pain in my body and in my mind.

This concentrates my attention very effectively. I have more unease and if I do not wise up to the situation the unease may develop into disease. I have been warned. I go back to the tribal doctor. He explains that I have a natural and constant balancing momentum and mechanism in my body working towards health. This mechanism aims at this balanced state of homeostasis. If I continue to force myself into chronic *overstress* my body's innate wisdom will make the decisions for me. The tribal doctor explains that if I continue my present lifestyle I could find my nervous systems at war with each other. They are both very powerful.

The power of the instinctive drive of the vegetative system is primitive. Its intention is to maintain life...and it is mindless. There is a volcano of undischarged emotion threatening to rise up from the body depths. To control this powerful explosive energy the central nervous system instructs the musculature to clamp down on the upsurge of the emotional strength. The diaphragm lies transversely across the middle of the body and influences, even controls, everything above and below it. In the startle reflex pattern I stop breathing. Its nerve supply is both voluntary and involuntary. Both vegetative and central nervous systems contribute to its functioning. This is a potential conflict area.

The central nervous system and the concept of Freud's 'ego' are interdependent. The ego meeting the deeper primitive body mechanisms is where the ego meets the other Freudian concept, the 'id'. The conscious meets the unconscious. It is a potential meeting of the titans. For a time, one or the other will be the stronger. The strength of the muscular ego will win. The muscle systems have clamped down on the vegetative system and the instinctive drives. This is an emotional repression. Gerda Boyesen calls this the somatic compromise. The drive towards homeostasis and balance is, however, always active and the power structures may not retain their power imbalances indefinitely.

I decide that I need another talk with the tribal doctor. I have an assortment of discomforts, which are becoming disturbing pains. The doctor asks me to say which of the painful discomforts is the worst. That is easy. I have a pain in my neck, which wakes me up at night and my face hurts, particularly around my eyes...and I have a stuffy nose. I tell the doctor about my problems with my neighbour and how I am feeling, not ill, but not well either. He suggests that we talk about this and that some informed touch therapy might help the discomforts in my body. A next possible step...and I now know who is the pain in my neck. This is the fifth stage.

Rehabilitation through therapeutic intervention

The word therapy comes from the Greek word '*therapaea*' which means 'service', 'being with', or 'attending'. It does not mean 'doing things to'. What I am about to recount is a biodynamic experience which will be a mixture of having attention paid to me and having things done to me.

29

The ancient Greeks did a lot of touch therapy and there are traces of the evidence below the Acropolis in Athens and other sites.

An account of my treatment

I lay down on the treatment table. The touch therapist and I talked a little. I told her about my present situation and what the tribal doctor had prescribed. The treatment session lasted about fifty minutes. The most dramatic part of the experience came when the therapist's fingertips were resting on the area of my cheeks below my eyes. My eyes were closed and I was aware of tensions in the tissues of my face, pain in my neck and some tenseness in my jaw and deep within my throat. Suddenly I experienced the beginnings of tiny vibrations around and below my eyes. They were very subtle and they suffused the whole of my face. They began to move down to my throat. This experience lasted for probably less than a minute.

For the first time I understood what words like 'streamings' and 'vegetative currents' and 'facial mask' meant. Other things happened in quick succession. I began to take deep breath releases one after another. I heard and felt rumblings from my belly. The tremblings in my face grew less but I felt a fizzy sensation throughout my body right down to my toes. I had a feeling of powerful wellbeing. There was significance in the increased sounds from my gut, which I had not been aware of at the beginning of the treatment session.

The history of Gerda Boyesen's theory of why these sounds appear is an extraordinary one. It remains a phenomenal factor in the biodynamic theory and philosophy. However cell biologists are finding that it may not be phenomenonological for much longer. Gerda Boyesen observed that when she was using physiotherapeutic skills on patients suffering from psycho-neurotic problems in their bodies, many things could happen to them.

After a treatment session involving special physiotherapeutic techniques, there were often after effects and vegetative responses. The patients could experience perspiration, an increase in urinary output, crying, vomiting and/or diarrhoea...and sometimes excessive shivering and trembling. The discharge of body fluids was very common. These symptoms could occur over some days, and accompanying these symptoms there were increases in the peristaltic sounds, the belly sounds mostly considered as relating to the sounds of digestion.

In addition to these observations Gerda Boyesen noticed that over the days and weeks following the release symptoms the patients remarked on feelings of well being and reductions in the severity of their psycho-neurotic symptoms. Sometimes the symptoms went away entirely. Because the bowel sounds appeared as a response to the therapeutic touch and were synonymous with psychological changes in the patient's overall condition; and they appeared to have no direct connection with food digestion, Gerda Boyesen called this peristaltic activity the 'secondary function' of the digestive tract, the 'psycho-peristalsis'.

She went on to describe this function of the digestive tract as the 'manifestation' of our deepest being – the unconscious. Gerda called the gut, the 'id canal'. Both Freud and Reich had looked for physical evidence of the unconscious but had not found it.

As a result of my therapeutic encounter with the biodynamic therapist I began to have valuable insights. The feeling of wellbeing lasted for about three days. Though the bliss did not last it had given me something to remember. My misery was not permanent. I would have to find alternative ways of dealing with threatening neighbours. For instance I could look for elements in my life that would provide opportunities to enhance the feeling of wellbeing. It is my birthright after all. In biodynamic psychology and philosophy the definition of the wellbeing is libido. Even the Oxford English Dictionary relates this to sexuality!

According to the Gerda Boyesen philosophy, libido is a function of the life force in its own right and not solely with respect to the sexual drive. There are many important questions still to be answered. One of them is where does all that fluid come from? What are the mechanisms in the body that deal with the battles between the nervous systems? What exactly occurs in the body when total attention is paid to another person? Does the electricity in the body have news for us? And so on...All need clarification and explanation.

The cat will, as far as we know, refuse to behave in a human way with all of the aggravation of being human. I do, however, know of a Burmese cat, which became completely bald when its family put it into kennels while they went house hunting for some months. The cat's fur grew again when the family was reunited.

CHAPTER 2

Self help for angina sufferers

What is angina?

Angina is not a disease in itself. It is an indication that something is seriously amiss and a consultation with the family doctor is the first thing on
the list of priorities. So many people go on and on, putting off the good
hard look at the way they are treating their bodies and very often denying
that there are clear and painful signals telling them that the time has
come to change the situation.

If you experience any of these symptoms, you must consult your
doctor. This material does not suggest any alternative to proper medical
attention. The correct term for the pain peculiar to the sufferer is angina
pectoris. It is derived from the Greek word 'agkhone', which means,
'strangled'. *Pectoris* is the Latin word for chest. There we have it!

What happens?

The pain may be dull or aching behind the breastbone. It sometimes
moves left across and down through the shoulder moving into the arm
and hand. Some sufferers feel the pain across the chest in both directions
and down both arms. Sometimes the pain travels up the side of the neck.
It may be a searing pain and breath taking, and it can be very alarming.
Sometimes it will appear after excessive effort or after some emotional
upheaval and it has a purpose. The most effective of its uses is to say
stop. It is also saying that the episode, which brought on the pain, may
have to be avoided next time.

The body has a very special wisdom, which is too often ignored by
the brain. When the body says 'stop', the brain intelligence will often say
'I must just finish this job and then I will listen to what my body is saying'. The body, however, is very fed up with being ignored. It eventually
makes a pain that really hurts. The body knows best and stops moving. I

have seen a person suffering from angina put a hand to the middle of the chest and then collapse to the floor. The legs have refused to work any more and lying or sitting has become the automatic response. It becomes painful and difficult to breathe and the chest becomes rigid – the shoulders are hunched and drawn forward in a movement that protects the front of the chest. Now the brain has to listen!

There are many theories about heart conditions and what causes the diseases of the arteries and heart. Theories are of small comfort to the person suffering from angina when the pain strikes; and fortunately there is always the pill or the capsule prescribed by the doctor to get the pain under control. Inside the chest the active drug in the pill or capsule relieves the tightened arteries. It is a tremendous comfort and relief to know that by carrying pills or capsules there is an available relief for the times of extreme discomfort and pain.

Let us look, though, at the immediate response of the body to the chest pain. Mostly, both hands go quite instinctively to the area of pain. However there is hardly ever time to watch what is happening. On the other hand there is, often, quite a lot of time in the day when there is no disabling pain. I would like you to think about this pain-free time and to use it, whenever and wherever it is possible. Believe that with regular attention and concentration on the chest wall and the left arm during the pain-free times you can make these pain-free times last longer. By your own caring for your body, you may reduce the frequency of the angina pectoris.

What to do

Take time off now to sit down in a firm, comfortable chair. Sit with your tail tucked comfortably into the back of the chair and sit as comfortably as you can. Remember that this can be enjoyable. Angina sufferers tend to have few real, pleasurable experiences in their bodies. There is often the ever-present fear of another attack. Sit with your legs slightly separated and comfortably supported by your unshod, uncrossed feet resting on a cushion or folded blanket. If the chair has arms, all the better. Let your arms rest wherever they feel most at ease.

Open and close your fists slowly and very luxuriously, stretch out your fingers and thumbs as far as they will go and then relax. Do this a few times and feel the difference as the warm blood reaches the nails and finger tips. Think of where your hands reach for when you have had a pain in your chest. Put your left hand, lightly, on that place. It may be somewhere in or behind your breastbone. Then put your right hand over your navel, just lightly. Breathe gently and normally, there is no need to take big deep breaths. You may, however, soon find you want to yawn or give a big sigh. Just let it happen. This is your own do-it-yourself relaxation.

You can do this any time you want to. You can do it almost anywhere, even when you are sitting on the loo! Just stay quietly like this breathing in and out gently, no deep breaths unless they come effortlessly by themselves. The next time you breathe out, let your shoulders relax and drop. Do this a few more times while you feel how you have been keeping your shoulders raised and tense for a long time.

When you have got used to the new feeling you may like to be a little more courageous. The next time you breathe out push your shoulders downward towards your seat. Take it gently and try not to hold your breath. Then relax! In a little while move your left hand down to the bottom of the ribs. Leave your right hand resting on the tummy over the navel. Breathe away gently, feeling the tensions loosen.

What your body wants

It is quite possible for you to feel like nodding off and have forty winks at this point. Then do just that! Your body never lies. If you nod off it is because your body needs it. Feel if there is anything that could make this experience just a little more comforting: perhaps a small cushion in the small of your back would be the thing; perhaps the room is too hot or too cool or too noisy.

Pleasure is important in relaxation. Sometimes there are intrusions that disturb your new-found tranquillity. You can only do your best and try to accept the imperfections!

Little and often

Do these small enjoyable things as often as you can. Stay with the peaceful things you have found yourself through your own efforts, for as long as you can. It is the beginning of the natural healing process in your body.

Help from family and friends

There are things that the family and friends can do if you are overtaken by an angina attack. Take your medically subscribed drug in the right dose. Sit or lie in the position which feels most comfortable. Wife, husband, friend or whoever is calm and caring may place themselves at the left-hand side of the person suffering.

1. Their right hand goes lightly on the sufferer's left shoulder and a very gentle pressure downwards is put on the joint. Each time there is a breathing out, press down gently in time with the breath. The pressure must be comforting rather than demanding that the shoulder should submit.

2. At the same time, the friend's left hand can rest lightly on the sufferer's left hand from wrist to finger, right to the finger ends and just lightly.

3. Stay like that quietly – as relaxed as possible while the pain is subsiding.

4. Stroking very gently from the tip of the shoulder on the left side down to the ring finger and little finger is effective and also gives the friend the feeling that some comfort is being given. This treatment is best done over the clothes for the simple reason that when an attack of angina comes, undressing is the last thing the person suffering needs.

If another person is there and wants to help, it is very comforting to have the feet held, lightly. Stroke gently from the ankles to the ends of the toes. Do not try to pick the feet up. Let them lie as they are but help the relaxation by gentle caring and stroking.

5. Sometimes the person suffering finds him or herself alone after the attack of pain has passed. When able, it is good to use the right hand to stroke the left arm down from the shoulder tip to the outside of the left

hand. Pull each finger, not forgetting the thumb, very gently. Stroke and pull and feel the pressure in the chest subside. Stay in the position of maximum ease for as long as possible.

Forget the job waiting to be done. Jobs do have a habit of waiting around looking impatient. The chances are that a sympathetic friend may see your anxiety and help out. So there is no great hurry to get back into circulation. It is also a time to reflect that maybe you are one of those people who pride themselves on not asking for help. Your pride is more important than your need for rest. Think about it!

High blood pressure

You may be suffering from or having treatment for high blood pressure. Remember that relaxation in one part of the body will bring some relaxation in all of the body so you are helping those tight muscles in the arteries to let go a little. You are sure to recognise that you have been uptight for a long time. Gently and often is the key to the success of relaxation.

The role of anger

When I work with patients who experience angina pain or who have high blood pressure, I often find that one of the most difficult things to deal with is the emotion of anger. When one is ill and worried and depressed it is really very hard to stay cool and calm. It is easy to feel irritated and angry over small things. It seems that tolerance of the small and insignificant episodes of the daily round gets less and less. Members of the family often guard themselves against the irritability of the heartsick patient.

Communication between members of even a loving family can become strained, even to breaking point. I know that it is said that we should not bottle up this anger. For the patient sick at heart, this can bring a dilemma. Do I lose my temper and express my rage even if it hurts the other person or persons? Or do I swallow my anger and, at the same time, deny that I am angry.

Unfortunately, few heartsick people realise how much they are denying their bodies any recognition. They say 'Oh! I'm all right. Stop fussing' or 'Yes! Of course I'm all right to go to work'. And they will go on denying their body right up to admission into the intensive care unit of the hospital's cardiac ward. Each time you indicate to your body that you understand what it is trying to say to you, by, for instance, giving you a bad pain in your chest, the more grateful it is and the more you help with your own healing process.

How to feel the anger

Fortunately, the body does offer an alternative. It takes a bit of courage but not as much as facing the results of the destructive courage, which says you're OK and hates fussing! First of all there is the feeling of anger, which rises from the pit of the belly up to the mouth. Something very small can release an enormous amount of rage. The next time this happens to you and you feel the anger rising, change the pattern. It will take a bit of courage, but you will soon learn how it works...after the first attempt. Ignore everybody and everything. Go quietly into the garden or somewhere else in the house.

Feel the anger. Take a breath and allow the feeling to go right through you and get in touch with how your arms and legs feel. Sometimes you will find that you are shaking. Good! Go on being aware of your breathing and the shaking. Just shake and feel the shaking. Hang on to something while this is happening. You may find that you have taken a deep spontaneous breath of release. You feel warm and relieved, and goodness me! You no longer feel enraged.

What you have done is to contain your anger and let it work for you instead of against you. You have not said or done things you may later regret. You have not produced any guilty feelings inside yourself. As a big bonus you may have saved yourself a bout of angina pain. You are not a saint, so do not expect to get the hang of all this in one go! You have been pretending to yourself and everybody else that you are a well and controlled person. You have been doing this for many a long day.

However, you have forgotten one important thing. Your body does not lie...even though your head lies. Sooner or later this must sink in to your know-all brain and the truth must be accepted. It's a funny thing, though, the more often you admit and learn to feel how angry you are, the less angry you become. This is a way to health for the heartsick patient. It could be the beginning of a new sort of life...if you care to try it.

CHAPTER 3

Communication, Intention and Attention – an essay[1]

Recently I was treating a young woman. She was suffering from a bowel disorder of ten years duration. Her history clearly indicated that the condition began after she had had a miscarriage at the beginning of her marriage when she was 19 years old. It was after the miscarriage that the bowel symptoms developed.

During the session she lay over on her left side in comfort. My left hand lay lightly at the junction of her cervical and thoracic spine. My right hand was resting lightly over the front of her thoracic cage, just over the diaphragm. I listened to the dry electric sounds alternating with loud bubbling water sounds. After about ten minutes of just being with this gentle holding, she said, 'What are you doing? I can feel funny sparkles down my arms and legs!'. After a slight pause she said, 'are you really a healer? – Your hands are so hot!'.

I knew a lot about this girl. I knew when she started to be ill, I knew what she had told me about her uncomfortable symptoms, I knew about her medication. I knew about her family and some of the problematic interactions in the family, I had a fair idea of what was going on in her bowel, inside and outside. I knew that she had told me she would do anything to get well. I actually touched this girl for less than fifteen minutes.

From experience I knew that a very little of this contact can do a great deal. For the rest of the session, one hour exactly, she rested. 'I feel deeply relaxed', she said later. In the following days she had an exacerbation of her symptoms and she released a lot of fluid and blood. How could touching her lightly for 15 minutes produce all this reaction? This is the perennial and ever present question.

---

1   This chapter was originally published as an article in the *Journal of Biodynamic Psychology*, Volume 3, Biodynamic Psychology Publications, London, 1982.

Ebba Boyesen's article in the *Journal of Biodynamic Psychology*[2] echoed many of my own cognitive and developing questions about therapy in general, and about myself. What is the contact and interaction between two people in the daily situation of therapy?

This patient's question about my being a healer is also relevant. Since I know that any healing which takes place is in the body mechanisms of the individual being treated, and not the result of healing rays which come from my hands, I question the assumption that many people make – 'I have something wrong with me, you heal me and make me better'.

There is, nevertheless, the most extraordinary situation in the British National Health Service at the moment where spiritual healing would be permitted in 1500 hospitals in this country if there were a request for it by a patient and if the relevant medical team were agreeable. This state of affairs must have an apt significance even though it may be used by patients, relatives and friends as a last-resort phenomenon.

I believe that there is in all therapy (*Therapaea* – Greek for 'tend') an amalgam of Communication, Intention and Attention. In the case I have just described there was a very good level of communication and I contributed the attention and intention in my work with her. Professor Dolores Krieger in her book *Therapeutic Touch*[3] uses the word 'Intentionality'. It is a prerequisite for success with the use and application of therapeutic touch. I shall come back to this later in my essay.

Communication

In looking at Communication, let us first look at the simplest form of life, the single cell organism of the amoeba. There is an outer permeable membrane. Contained within the membrane is the cytoplasmic fluid and an inner nucleus. The nucleus contains the genetic information which governs its function. It is a simple, single, self-sufficient organism. In order that it can live, it takes in through its outer membrane carbohy-

---

2   Boyesen. Ebba, 'The Essence of Therapy', *Journal of Biodynamic Psychology*, Volume 2, Biodynamic Psychology Publications, London, 1981.
3   Kreiger, Dolores, *Therapeutic Touch*, Englewood Cliffs NJ, Prentice Hall, 1979.

drates, protein and fat. What it does not need it excretes in the opposite direction.

When it reaches its optimum size, regulated by directions from the nucleus instruction centre, it splits into two. The nucleus, itself, divides and the cytoplasm follows the new individual nuclei and each new little cell becomes enclosed in a new outer membrane. The process results in there being two new cells. This is the innate genetic pattern of cell division in the amoeba. It is this movement of expansion and contraction and momentum that gives direction following the genetic instructions from the nucleus, that is the difference between a live cell and a dead cell. These are the basic patterns of life. The amoeba is a very simple and uncomplicated organism and is limited in potential. It is an independent entity so that communication between one amoeba and another is not apparently necessary.

However the human organism is made up of a great number of cells. Whilst there is a similar pattern of functioning to that of the amoeba, there is an inter-functioning between them that is extremely complex. The evolutionary leap from this simple organism to the vastly complicated human organism is huge. The basic biological laws, however, still operate. Providing there is the life energy to produce the movement and momentum then the human organism or any other organism will work with varying degrees of efficiency.

It is on the basic pattern of cell functioning that the Gerda Boyesen theory and its practical application depends. The cells of the human organism are basically of the same pattern as the amoeba. The evolution of the human being through the cell's adaptation to the needs of the evolving human being has resulted in the myriad of varieties, types, shapes and functions of cells. The organisation of cells into systems with separate but interdependent functions is the miracle of human life as we experience it.

In the application of the Gerda Boyesen theory to somatic and psychopathology it is thus inherent in the ethic of the approach that it is at the cell and system level that we view the human being. It is through the understanding that there is a most complex communication within the human organism, that it is possible to influence changes where the normal functioning has broken down and degrees of unease or disease in the psyche or soma have occurred. It is a gigantic task. For example, most medical students find that a textbook on human physiology is out of date by the time the first chapter has been researched and written. New conclusions relating to human biological functioning are emerging almost daily.

The minutiae of nerve cell function research is one example. It is very difficult to find hard evidence on the actual function of the nerve cells in the parasympathetic distribution. Unpublished work in this area of the vegetative system seems to show identifiable ganglia in the skin tissue where none was known previously. We have our suspicions, daily, that the right contact on the right skin area appears to counteract the effects of chronic sympathetic nervous activity. This touch is a form of direct communication and is an essential factor in the therapeutic process.

From empirical evidence, Gerda Boyesen developed the phenomenological concept of reduction in the chronic over-arousal of the sympathetic nervous system, which is monitored in her biodynamic work through a stethoscope placed on the belly. The question is, how does this happen? How does the contact of skin on skin (and very often the two skins are separated by clothing) produce such far-reaching reactions in the depths of the organism?

Going back to the amoeba for a moment, the apparent simplicity of the cell function is perhaps not so simple. That very self-contained way in which the amoeba goes about its business is, I think, a bit suspect for a simple organism. It is as though, in a most philosophical way, it knows its place. It may not be enough to say that all its life instructions are there in the nucleus and that it cannot go wrong. It may be very aware of its environment and when there is an awareness of the environment there is also the strong possibility of there being a connection and a communication. There is also the direction of the instruction from the nucleus. This complex structure contains something like a contracted, concentrated memory. The survival of the amoeba depends on the interpretation of the old learned facts.

To what end is the genetic computer directed? It is towards life. The interaction of the environment and the genetic apparatus involves a communication in order that life should continue. The very complexity of the body of a human being needs a library to store all the facts about it. The systems are comparatively easy to separate into the skeletal system, the muscular, the cardiovascular, the lymphatic, the nervous, digestive, urinary, endocrine, reproductive systems and the skin. There are billions of living, dying and dead cells in the human body at any given moment. They are all contained in the systems, and the general pattern is that each cell knows its place and function and each cell behaves accordingly (on the whole). When there is an aberration, then certain arrangements are made to try to put things straight – this is what has been called homeostasis.

In order that a good communication system can work, it is necessary to have a definitive organisation with which to communicate. It is a two-way process. It is also a dynamic process. It is possible to take the human being apart; to describe with some accuracy the various systems that make up the whole, together with the known functions of the systems; and yet; to miss altogether, the essence of the human being. The *gestalt* of a person is important in that the whole is greater than the sum of the parts; the human being is something more than an amalgamation of the various systems.

Case Discussion

Let us consider Gerda Boyesen's treatment of Oscar,[4] the patient with manic depressive psychosis, and the subsequent harmony of Oscar's pathological state. This treatment and approach was the result of Gerda's insight into the similarity or the amoebic energetic response and the pathological non-function of the total complexity of the cells making up Oscar's organism.

Gerda communicated her understanding of the abnormality of Oscar's living. She reached through to the contraction and expansion of cell function and followed the path of the life energy pattern. Oscar's internal communication system was badly disrupted and needed an external understanding, an external awareness and a communication of both in order that he could move towards his potential for normal functioning. In the treatment there was an internal communication as Oscar had his insights.

---

4   Boyesen, Gerda, Case History of a Manic-Depressive, in *Collected Papers of Biodynamic Psychology*, Volumes 1 and 2, Biodynamic Psychology Publications, London, 1969-79.

There was the external communication from Gerda that reached through to cell level.

It was at cell level that Oscar began his long haul out of the abyss. Gerda's treatment was at first directed towards the correction of the disturbed cellular mechanism of contraction-expansion-discharge. Then a vast realignment of inter- and extra-cellular content was set in motion. The totality of the Oscar organism underwent changes of great complexity on all levels...changes that involved latent time-scale stasis. For instance, the regression to very early disturbances in development demonstrated the optimistic fact that such stasis need not be permanent. The Oedipal development was seriously damaged and he got very stuck in the time scale reference.

Gerda's communication demonstrated the optimistic fact that such stasis need not mean permanent damage to the organism. The organismic logic is there, in the systems and in the cells. The logic of the body is undeniable. It is with this logic that we learn to communicate and at this point we must also understand some of the logic of the gestalt of the organism. As psychotherapists we actively train and promote the undoing processes of our own illogicalities. However we have no logical blueprint from which to work. When we contemplate the inference that everything follows a pattern that is predictable and without variation, we move into an altogether different area. Modern physics and philosophy offer little comfortable predictability. There are no straight lines. There are no firm conclusions. However the questions will not go away.

When I began to write this essay, I was bothered by the nagging feeling that sooner or later, I would have to ask the physicists to answer some of these questions. Neurophysiology is a developing discipline and too far away from the researching going on in physics. It still remains locked into the minutiae. The cosmic view is an anathema. Embryology has too many 'don't knows'. Still, progress is being made, and in mammalian embryology it is possible to make hypotheses. It is possible to perceive possible connections and possible communications between parts of the body quite remote from each other. There is a subtlety beyond the present knowledge of physiology. The need to ask questions directs our perceptions. When enough perceptions have been made and appear to hold together through experience and verification of the results, it is then possible to make the concept.

It still remains in the area of phenomenalism, however. This train of thought follows a well-known phenomenon, well known to practitioners of biodynamic psychology at least. For example, I would perhaps be directing my therapeutic attention to a patient's left shoulder. The stethoscope indicates a response with release sounds. The patient takes a big release breath. Suddenly there is a flash of pain or awareness in my own left shoulder. My response to this phenomenon is to let it go. I feel that this is not my experience on the essential level. It is a cognitive experience, but it is a second-hand experience.

Sometimes the second-hand experience is of a sudden, sharp anxiety feeling. There is no obvious reason why this sharp anxiety should be there, it sometimes gets caught in my diaphragm and I have to leave the room, wash my hands, center myself, release my diaphragm by whatever means is appropriate and return to the patient. Sometimes the patient will say 'I felt as though I let something go!' and sometimes I confirm that something did indeed go. It depends on the immediate situation whether or not I make this confirmation and give a verbal feedback. This kind of experience is not at all rare and many people have similar tales to tell. So it seems that there is some form of communication happening.

The important point for me to remember is that the dynamic towards homeostasis that is manifesting itself in the patient belongs to the patient and not to me. I do not hold within myself the dynamic undoing process. For one thing my cell frequency is unique to me and the patient's cell frequency is unique to him or her. In general, the activity going on in the patient should dissipate into thin air or somewhere, if I do act as a kind of channel of release. But why did I feel the awareness in my left shoulder and where is this feeling?

I postulate, but cannot prove, that there is a remote memory in the cell area and body configuration of the shoulder, of some recognition that my shoulder and the patient's shoulder share a memory. I am trying, in the therapeutic sense, to stay with the experience the patient is having and not to get bogged down in the cognitive awareness of what is happening to me. I repeat, at this point, that I knew that I needed some stimulating guidance from physics or some other relevant discipline.

One morning the postman delivered a parcel of books that I had sent on ahead of me as I left Australia. The parcel contained Arthur

Koestler's *Janus – A Summing Up*,[5] Hans Selye's *The Stress of Life*[6] and Marilyn Ferguson's *The Aquarian Conspiracy*.[7] I opened the Koestler book and read:

> Jung's Essay on Synchronicity published in 1952 was partly based on Paul Kammerer's book, *Das Gesetz der Serie*, published in 1919. Kammerer was the brilliant Viennese experimental biologist of Lamarckian persuasion, who was accused of faking his results and who committed suicide in 1926 at the age of forty-five.
> He was throughout his life fascinated by co-incidences and from the age of 20-40 years kept a logbook of them...as Jung did.

Over the page I read:

> Kammerer said...'We thus arrive at the image of a world mosaic or cosmic kaleidoscope, which, in spite of constant shufflings and rearrangements also takes care of bringing like and like together!'

This gives me an insight into what was happening in my shoulders. I am, by this time, more than a little aware of the concept of Synchronicity (Jung) or Seriality (Kammerer). Kammerer calls it a Law that goes way beyond phenomenalism. It is Kammerer's Law of Seriality. I quote again from Koestler:

> Kammerer expresses his belief that Seriality is ubiquitous and continuous in Life, Nature and Cosmos. It is the umbilical cord that connects thought, feeling, science and art with the womb of the Universe, that gave birth to them.

All this ties in with what 1 believe to happen in my Communication with my patients. Once, Fritjof Capra, the author of the *Tao of Physics*[8] was speaking on the radio. He said that today, astro and nuclear physicists believe there is a connection between all sub-atomic particles in the universe. Furthermore in 1550 the early Renaissance Philosopher, Pico Della Mirandola wrote,

---

5   Koestler, Arthur, *Janus – A Summing Up*, Pan Books, 1979.
6   Selye, Hans *The Stress of Life,*
7   Ferguson, Marilyn, *The Aquarian Conspiracy*, Paladin, 1982.
8   Capra, Fritjof, *The Tao of Physics,* Flamingo 3rd Edition, 1982.

Firstly there is the unity in things whereby each thing is at one with itself, consists of itself and coheres with itself. Secondly, there is the unity whereby one creature is united with the others and all parts of the world constitute one world.[9]

There is, it would seem, a better chance of finding the answers to Biodynamic Psychology questions about Communication amongst the physicists and philosophers than in the current books of physiological findings.

Intention and Attention

Communication at a subtle level seems to be more of a possibility than it did at the beginning of this essay, but what about the concepts of Intention and Attention? The attention given to another human being would seem to be the first priority. There are no assumptions here; it is a cognitive activity. I focus my being on the moment as it is. Therapist and patient are spatially apart. Whatever is happening to the patient, all that the therapist can properly do is to attend. Which is where we came in earlier. ('*Therapaea*'...Greek for 'tend' and 'attend' meaning 'tend to'). No therapy can take place unless the therapist attends to the client.

The success of biodynamic therapy is that we do not just attend to what the client says or brings to the session, nor just to the symptoms or the changes in the breathing pattern, skin colour and tone, etc. within the process of the session. We attend to the whole person and aim to be with the patient in the totality of their organism.

Gerda Boyesen frequently says that one cannot touch one part of a person without touching the whole person, and this concept can be extended further. It is no news that the subtleties of the live organism reach beyond the confines of the skin. Some people see this communication area, others just feel it, and many can sense it. There are questions being asked as to its exact constitution. Some appear to have been answered by explanations within the realms of electricity and/or magnetism. We certainly use the concept of this communication area in our work. We postulate that life energy moves in and out and through the skin. We say it moves up and down, inside and outside the body. If it does not then we

9   Quoted in Koestler, Arthur, *Janus – A Summing Up,* Pan Books, 1979.

are dead. I have no knowledge of the forces of this subtle area being tested, but when there is a problem of cessation of vital functions the doctor asks him- or herself: 'Is this person really dead?'

There seems little doubt now that something which can be seen by the naked eye by some, and which can be photographed by others for those who are not able to see, surrounds any organism. There is evidence that the inorganic may also have a similar corona or aura. Exactly what happens in this subtle outside field is still speculative. If, however, the camera does not lie and the eyes of certain people are trustworthy, then it seems to be possible to say that there are sub-atomic particles moving and making what seems to be light. I have had the experience of seeing rapidly disappearing trails of what looked like light leaving my fingertips when I have been massaging a patient. It would be a very hazardous journey through laboratory tests, should I feel it necessary to prove what I think I saw.

The physicists say that in the realm of the electron and the atom, atoms are not things. The electrons that form an atom's shells are no longer 'things' in the sense of classical physics. When we get down to the atomic level, the objective world in space and time no longer exists.[10] All this is very dangerous ground from which to take a debate. There is no harm, though, in making an hypothesis in the special area of biodynamic experience.

Let me go on to the assumption that if there is one person in a life energy field producing movement on the sub-atomic level in another person's energy field, part of that dynamic may come from extra electrical movement caused by the cognitive apparatus, the central nervous system. The therapist makes the cognitive decision to attend to this totality. Professor Dolores Krieger[11] found that when she was conducting experiments with the technique using nursing staff and patients, the effective nurse was the nurse who felt compassion for the patient. These experiments were verified in a laboratory setting. There were significant changes in levels of haemoglobin in the subject's blood when compassion was put into the experimental situation. These experiments shed some light on what she called the 'interactional zone' between therapist and patient.

10   Quoted in Koestler, Arthur, *Janus – A Summing Up*, Pan Books 1979.
11   Krieger, Dolores, Therapeutic *Touch*, New York, 1981.

This is an area into which intent can be introduced after attention has been paid. It is probably the area where the effective therapist is most effective. The mandatory cleansing process of sorting out the illogicalities within the therapist using biodynamic psychology techniques is part of the biodynamic training programme and the value of this cleansing process is obvious. It seems even more obvious if the importance of objectivity is a criterion for an effective therapist. It certainly does not end at the end of the training programme. It is a process of cleansing, learning and knowing. No sooner has one clear insight emerged from the continuum of the dynamic process than another, even deeper, level develops and has to emerge, and so it goes on. It is a dynamic development process always bringing continuing insight.

Robert St. John's work with Prenatal Therapy[12] emphasises the importance of what is in the interactional zone. In his work he says it is necessary not to get involved on an emotional level with the person's struggle towards perfection. In biodynamic work we know this and we have a better chance of avoiding the hazards of disturbing the dynamic. Perhaps the intent that is put into the interactional zone functions on the sub-atomic level and could explain why some therapists report that, after giving a massage they feel expanded. Perhaps there is as much reorganisation and realignment going on at this level in the therapist as in the patient.

This week I have to see the physician who cares for the patient I began this essay with. I am not very optimistic about the communication we are likely to have. He does not believe in acupuncture or any of the health food fads. I think I will have to resort to putting a good dose of compassion into the interactional zone that will certainly be there between us. Herbert Spencer,[13] the English philosopher once wrote

> Mankind never tries the right remedy until it has exhausted every possible wrong one and there is a principle which is against all argument and which cannot fail to keep a man in everlasting ignorance. That principle is condemnation without investigation.

I conclude that the relative importance of Communication, Intention and Attention is hard to establish. That all three are vitally important in ef-

---

12   St. John, Robert, *Metamorphosis,* London, 1978.
13   Spencer, Herbert, *Principles of Biology,* London, 1872.

fective therapy I have stated previously. I believe Gerda Boyesen's work gives us the means to get insights that help us use these concepts effectively and extend our understanding of others and ourselves as human beings.

CHAPTER 4

The biodynamic approach to causes and treatment of idiopathic lower back pain[1]

Pain in the back has reached epidemic proportions. An extract from the report of the *Federation Internationale de Medecin* presented to the International Congress held at Kensington Town Hall, London, 18-22 September 1989, revealed currently known figures and statistics.

Mr. Peter Apsley, the Executive Director of the National Back Pain Association was invited to present the economics of back pain. In his introduction he said that back pain is amongst the most common causes of absenteeism from work...and that it may well be the most common cause. In the United Kingdom, Department of Health and Social Security figures showed that 46.5 million working days were lost through back pain in the financial year 1987-88, i.e. 12% of all days lost through illness.

The Office of Health Economics estimates the cost to British Industry at rather more than two billion pounds per annum. Figures published in the *Lancet* suggest that the United States of America loses an estimated 217 million working days each year at a cost to the country's economy of as much as 11 trillion dollars per annum. The statistics relating to the back pain sufferers are by no means the whole story. The effects reach out to family as well as employers. Peter Apsley reported that

> The children of back pain sufferers cried and whined, complained of sickness and were absent from school thrice as often as children in the other group...like their fathers, these children felt excessively helpless at controlling their health.

Sexual relationships can be inhibited and social relationships can be disastrously affected and disturbed. Sporting and leisure activities are curtailed. Not infrequently, the pain and general life disturbance can lead to marriage break up and occasionally, suicide.

1   This chapter was first published as an article in 1989.

The orthodox medical model

Acute back pain will always be a condition that calls for expert medical attention. When the acutely painful and disabling stage has passed, but a chronic pain in a limb continues to plague the patient, the investigative procedures may extend to hospital departments. The special skills of the orthopaedic specialist, the neurologist, the gynaecologist and the psychiatrist may all be needed. If something is found, relevant to the painful condition, the appropriate treatment will follow and the patient will improve and begin to enjoy life once more. The potential causes of back pain are many and varied. They all need expert attention. Some could be life threatening.

Some of the causes of back pain

> Congenital bone deformities
> Tumours (benign or malignant)
> Inflammatory diseases such as rheumatoid arthritis
> Degenerative diseases such as osteoporosis
> Trauma
> Poor muscle tone following neurological damage, e.g. anterior poliomyelitis (Infantile paralysis)
> Chronic postural strain
> Pelvic disease such as uterine and ovarian conditions

The idiopathic lower back pain

An unknown percentage of people who seek help for their painful backs are told they have no discernible pathology that could account for their symptoms. The doctors have reassured them that there is no disease or damage and the patient is referred back from whence they came...back to the family doctor. The diagnosis of the patient who is declared free of disease, though not of dis-ease, is that it is an idiopathic back pain. Sometimes the patient may have symptoms of depression, feeling low, have poor sleep patterns, and not much appetite for anything.

Constant pain is depressing. It gets in the way of feeling well and free. When the patient has been reassured and told that there is no disease, there is a temporary lifting of the spirits. Many times, however, the old nagging pain returns, together with the depressing feelings of being trapped in a prison of hopelessness. This is depressing because the outlets from the prison are reduced by at least one. In all the hustle and bustle and the anticipation of a cure there can be confusion. The competent specialists have done all the necessary tests and found nothing to account for the pain. All is well, in fact...but the pain continues.

It may be that the patient has forgotten that well before the back pain struck they were feeling depressed; there was a feeling that life was being a bit harsh long before the first episode of pain. If the current depression deepens or persists, the family doctor may prescribe an anti-depressant and perhaps a mild hypnotic drug to regain any lost or disturbed sleeping pattern and this may work very well. If the medical attention does not succeed or reach the expectations of the sufferer, they may be tempted to seek help from a complementary source.

The biodynamic approach to the idiopathic back pain.

This category of the condition is idiopathic because it is not occasioned or preceded by another disease. If the patient seeks help from outside the orthodoxy of medicine they may chose a discipline from a range of concepts and techniques. Osteopathy, Chiropractic, Homeopathy, Acupuncture or the Alexander Technique and other disciplines are valuable. Biodynamic theory and practice are in this area of complementary disciplines. The focus of attention here is somewhat different from other disciplines. Although most of the effective concepts and techniques take the whole person into account there are fundamental differences.

The essential ingredient of the biodynamic approach to illness or to health for that matter comes from the insights of Gerda Boyesen. Her training in clinical psychology and physiotherapy provided the essential background for the development of her insights. Gerda Boyesen saw the psychoanalytical concepts of the ego and the id as having physical manifestations, which could be approached through the physical body. Other psychoanalysts, including Freud himself, had hypothesised that there must be physical evidence for the existence of the ego and the id but it was never identified.

The phenomenon of the gut having a secondary function was an important insight. The body needs a mechanism for the propulsion of food eaten for nutrition so that the mechanisms of metabolism can act. This mechanism is called peristalsis. Gerda Boyesen found that there was, in the central digestive canal, the gut, a secondary function other than the digestion of nutritional substances. This secondary function of the gut appeared to have an ability to digest the residual overstress elements in the body.

This secondary function of the gut, Gerda Boyesen called 'psycho-peristalsis'. From the point of view of scientific verification this function still remains in the category of the phenomenological. Practitioners of biodynamic techniques know that psycho-peristalsis is a trusted monitor of the way the human (not to mention the animal) being, maintains a constant struggle towards homeostasis and harmony. In order to hear this secondary function of the gut, a stethoscope is placed in the region of the lower abdomen.

The presenting symptoms of idiopathic lower back pain are communicating an important message to anyone prepared to listen. The biodynamic therapist acts as a companion in the therapeutic situation to the sufferer, while they both explore the route to the place from whence came the urgent message that someone should pay attention to what is wrong. They are helped along this journey in the knowledge that there is a dissolving and digesting mechanism which will deal with the old emotional traumas.

Perhaps, the pain of these old events will be understood and dissolved once and for all. The medical histories of many of the lower back pain sufferers reveal a range of common symptoms, although not necessarily at the same time. Recall of these symptoms often emerges later in the therapeutic process, the initial consultation having no mention and perhaps no memory of the symptoms.

Common symptoms

>   Chronic weariness
>   Depressive feelings
>   Insomnia
>   Stressful feelings

Bowel problems, for example, bouts of diarrhoea, constipation, bloating

A history of appendicitis, that settled down without surgery.

A history of appendicitis that needed surgery, after which the bowel problems improved but there was a recurrence of episodic back pain.

The journey towards an hypothesis

In Australia I led a group of health professionals in an introduction to biodynamic psychology weekend seminar. Included in the group were a number of senior chiropractors. They told me about the chiropractic approach to the Irritable Bowel Syndrome (IBS). This syndrome is a chronic, relapsing condition and involves a painful alternation of diarrhoea and constipation, which occurs episodically. The majority of these patients had found the condition easier to cope with when they had been investigated and found to be free from dangerous pathology. It is an idiopathic condition with a strong hypothesis that overstress may be involved.

Chiropractic recognises the condition as involving the ileo-caecal valve and calls it the ileo-caecal valve syndrome. Chiropractic splits the syndrome further into:

> The open ileo-caecal valve syndrome
> The closed ileo-caecal valve syndrome

The Open Ileo-Caecal Valve Syndrome

This syndrome presents symptoms of pain and diarrhoea and bed-rest is prescribed for relief. Cold, not iced, packs may be applied to the right-*iliac fossa* area of the lower abdomen. Diet may need some care and a bland diet is recommended. These steps will often afford relief of the symptoms. The chiropractor may use a physical approach to the problem and use kinesiology and muscle adjustment techniques in a special sequence. If the diarrhoea persists, the chiropractor may have to inflict a sharp shock impulse over the ileo-caecal valve area. For this manoeuvre he uses an instrument which behaves like a sophisticated pop gun and causes the ileo-caecal valve, which has no nerve supply, to contract and close off the opening into the caecum. This technique stops the diarrhoea more often than not.

The Closed Ileo-Caecal Valve Syndrome

This syndrome is associated with constipation and a spastic descending colon. Pain is constant or episodic as the symptoms ebb and flow. The chiropractor will often view the sufferer as being an uptight individual. The syndrome appears to correlate significantly with emotional and mental states. There may be disturbance in the blood sugar levels. Depression and anxiety are correlated significantly. The chiropractic treatment includes some supervision of diet and the reassurance that getting up from bed could ease the discomfort.

The Great Mimicker

There are so many observed symptoms occurring with the ileo-caecal valve that it has been called the great mimicker of disorders. The symptoms may occur singly or several may occur at the same time. The variety of symptoms includes: shoulder joint pain, sudden low back pain, pain round the heart, dizziness, flu symptoms, pseudo-bursitis, pseudo sacro-iliac strain, tinnitus, nausea, faintness, pseudo-sinus infection, pseudo-hyperchlorhydria, headache, sudden thirst, pallor, dark circles under the eyes and bowel disorders.

Case History

Still in Australia. The day after I had led the introduction to biodynamic psychology weekend, I received a telephone call from one of the participants of the weekend. Ann, a chiropractor, worked locally. She had a busy and successful practice. She was married with two grown up children. Ann told me she had a chronic pattern of episodic diarrhoea, pain in the abdomen and feelings of weariness. She was becoming worried about the reduction of the time interval between the symptoms.

58

As a practitioner she was well aware of what she should sensibly do. Her family doctor had arranged for her to have tests to evaluate any colonic damage or disease. The results were comforting up to a point. She was relieved that there were no signs of ulceration or malignancy. Two weeks after having received the welcome assurance that there was no pathology, she had another bout of diarrhoea and pain. A chiropractor colleague had treated her with the technique of administering a sharp shock impulse over the ileo-caecal valve area. The diarrhoea ceased for twelve hours and Ann rested and took a bland diet. Then the symptoms began again and it had affected her weekend.

Ann telephoned me for an appointment the day after the workshop. Apart from the obvious inconvenience, Ann was not unduly uncomfortable but she felt excessively tired...and she had a backache. With some reluctance I agreed to see her. I am not happy with one-off treatments under these circumstances and I was about to travel to another part of the country. On the other hand I had a very reputable colleague in the town who had had biodynamic experience and she would be careful with the treatment of Ann's condition. My reluctance to treat Ann and then to leave the area was due to an experience I had had on three occasions.

Another patient who was suffering from Irritable Bowel Syndrome lay over on her left side while I listened for the psycho-peristalsis. At first there were no sounds. Then, I placed my left hand over the cervical-thoracic junction and my right hand over the thoracic diaphragm and waited in this position for about ten minutes in order to give the psycho-peristalsis time to establish. This was the extent of the touch therapy.

No sounds came after this and the patient rested for the rest of the treatment session, still lying on her left side. After resting she dressed and left. A week later when she kept her second appointment she said she had had quite a lot of blood in her stool. This patient had never had bowel bleeding previously. My understanding of this was that even a very gentle touch could produce a strong parasympathetic response. This could result in the fragile epithelial lining of the gut, shredding.

A similar reaction to touch occurred in one patient suffering from a chronic depressive state and another patient whose emotional life was chaotic but needed help for a chronic lower back pain. The experiences caused me to be very wary of the resulting parasympathetic response when tissue had been chronically affected.

Ann's treatment session began with an interview lasting half an hour. She was feeling very tired, so the interview took place while she lay on the treatment table. I asked her how she thought I could help her. She began to talk. She told me about her recent medical history. She spoke about her fears that she was getting worse, and that she could develop some definite pathology. I agreed to treat her because the medical experts had so recently investigated her and found her to be free of bowel disease.

As she lay supine on the massage table I listened for any psycho-peristaltic sounds. Then I asked her to turn over on to her left side with her knees bent. I placed my right hand over the solar plexus and my left hand over the junction of the neck and thorax. There were no sounds. I remained in this position for fifteen minutes. At the end of this time there were a few intermittent watery sounds. She gave two or three release breaths and then appeared to be deeply relaxed. I removed my hands very gently and Ann rested for a further half-hour.

She got up from the table very slowly at the end of this time. We reviewed any changes she felt in her body. I saw that she looked very tired and was aware of her exhaustion. The next morning she telephoned to say that the diarrhoea had increased and that she had decided to stay in bed. She was not in pain but felt excessively weary. On the third day she was feeling much better and on the fourth day she passed a formed stool.

It was arranged that she should receive further biodynamic treatment from a colleague who had been informed of my findings. I received a report a month later, which indicated that Ann was feeling less exhausted. She said 'I have a better relationship with my gut and I understand my need to become exhausted'. She was having less pain and no diarrhoea and was passing formed stools.

The biodynamic theory applied to this disorder of the gut

The biodynamic theory and technique used in treating Ann was simple to use. However, the simplicity of the technique does not make it easy to understand the changes in physiology. The ileo-caecal valve lies between the terminal ileum and the caecum. It has no nerve supply but responds to pressure as the residual metabolic matter is pushed along by the metabolic peristalsis of the ileum. Ann's intestines were behaving abnormally. The question was how and why the abnormality arose.

An understanding of the Gerda Boyesen concept of visceral armour is crucial at this point. Life is full of emergencies, little and large, and the body responds in order to cope with the emergency. A stimulus (danger to the organism) causes an autonomic nervous response and as a result a charge of hormonal energy floods straight into the bloodstream. Adrenalin rushes to the muscular system through the blood supply and the organism is charged to flee or fight. For a short time in the alert state between stimulus and discharge of energy in fleeing or fighting, the maximum readiness to respond to the emergency is mobilised.

This surge of response causes intestinal contraction as well as, amongst other physiological responses, a musculo respiratory inhibition. It is meant to be a short-term physiological event and when the emergency is over and dealt with, all the physiological functions involving the conservation of energy can, and biologically should, relax, let go and return to normal. The intestinal activity passes from the sympathetic nervous influence to the parasympathetic. From energy movement upwards in the body towards expression, to downwards after the expressive action, into recovery and recuperation.

The hormonal response to danger

Stimulus	alert to danger.
Charge	preparation to carry out the action.
Action	discharge to expression.
Recuperation	recovery and the return of the readiness mechanisms back to normal.

If the charge is not completed and the discharge is not fully expressed a chronic pattern of physiological change can result. In these circumstances therapeutic intervention may be indicated. In the rehabilitation stage various therapeutic techniques may be needed. For a short period in the alert stage between charge and discharge of energy into action there is a closure, containment pattern in the intestinal tract. If the organism does not complete the emotional cycle into the recuperative stage and after hundreds of similarly incomplete cycles have occurred, the closure pattern becomes a chronic state.

The result of this chronic condition is that the intestinal tissue does not pulsate healthily along its length. The emotional content of countless arousal patterns builds up into a chronic condition. The inefficient intestines will not pulsate and propel their contents because of the excess of fluid throughout the intestinal walls. This excess fluid is not accounted for in biological, physiological and scientific terms.

The explanation remains phenomenological but was defined by Wilhelm Reich in his Cosmic Laws 1 and 2.[2] Gerda Boyesen describes this fluid as 'chemostatic fluid', the fluid that according to Reich is the result of Cosmic Law 1. This Cosmic Law states that where there is a strong orgonotic or energy field, this field will attract water. The strong orgonotic or energy field in the gut is the result of the undischarged hormonal and emotional residue. This is a particular kind of fluid which is composed of water, plus the emotional and biochemical or hormonal residue. This is what Gerda Boyesen calls the chemostatic fluid.

This theoretical explanation for the disturbed function of the gut is not scientifically proven, but scientists in the field of New Science for example Fritzof Capra, David Bohm[3] et al. are softening the edges of the mechanistic approach to orthodox biology. With the continuing experiences and observations of constancy in the therapeutic results, some future enlightenment is inevitable. Unexplained and unwanted fluid is inherent in many psychosomatic conditions. It becomes more explicable when the theory of chemostatic fluid is interposed. The concept of chemostatic fluid explains the link with what was happening to Ann.

In the centre of the human organism there is a tube which takes in nourishment at one end and releases what is no longer of use to the organism at the other end. It has primitive origins in the worm from which it came. Gerda Boyesen calls this internal tube, with all its sophisticated development since it was a simple worm, the 'Id Canal'. This channel is where, in part, the physical manifestation of the unconscious lies.

Both Freud and Reich considered it more than possible that the unseen unconscious could be a reality in the flesh. Freud called his concept

2   Wilhelm Reich pursued his understanding of the power of the Cosmic Energy in 'Cosmic Orgone Energy and Ether'. *Orgone Energy Bulletin,* Vol. 1, No 4, 1949. Reich's Cosmic Laws are also discussed in Boyesen, Mona Lisa , 'Dynamics of the Vasomotoric Cycle', *Energy and Character*, Vol. 6, No. 2, 1975.

3   Weber, Renee, 'Conversations with David Bohm, Fritzof Capra', in *The Holographic Paradigm,* Shambala, 1982.

the *Id* (the instinctive drives). Groddeck called it the *It*[4] Pain of any kind is the alarm which alerts the individual that all is not well and that something is in need of attention.

Ann's pain was meant to do just that and the signals had only partially been heard. Her pain was a communication from the central nervous system that something needed to be done. This pain came from the nerve centres in the gut, which lie close to the inner lining. The involvement of the musculature was crucial to the need to remove the unwanted fluid and the re-establishment of a healthy peristalsis. Therefore there is a connection between the central nervous system, the muscular coats of the gut and that part of the gut which is the physical manifestation of the id.

The development of these three integrated elements is derived embryonically. The central nervous system and the skin, develop from the ectoderm. The muscular system of the body, including the abdominal muscles and the peristaltic muscles develop from the mesoderm. The innermost lining of the gut, the epithelial lining, develops from the endoderm. The blood supply to these tissues is, of course, partly arterial. The arteries and the tiny arterioles also have muscular coats and although it is not totally established that the whole of the inner lining, the epithelial lining, is developed from the endoderm, some of it is.

Note

Clinical experience of working with some patients suffering from high blood pressure, and clinically diagnosed as having arterio-sclerosis, who are being treated with drugs to reduce their clinical symptoms; recover from a high degree of pathology when biodynamic concepts and techniques are added to the treatment repertoire. A normo-tensive state may be achieved and maintained. It is obviously impossible to test the theory that this is so without extensive clinical research. There are many influences, which would have to be taken into account.

---

4   Groddeck, Georg, *The Book of the It,* NMD Publications Co., 1928.

The biology of the body fluids

Water makes up about 70% of the body weight. In a man weighing 70 kg. there will be about 45 litres of water in his body. Of this, 30 litres is termed intra-cellular. Outside the cells there are about 5 litres of extra-cellular fluid. The extra-cellular fluid is plasma from the blood and body tissues, called interstitial fluid or tissue fluid. The physiological formation of tissue fluid is important for the understanding of Gerda Boyesen's theory of chemostasis.

Blood flowing through blood vessels does not come into contact with cells of the body. It stays in the blood vessels. The nearest blood vessel to a cell is the capillary. The space between the capillary and the cell is filled with fluid, tissue fluid. Nutrients and oxygen have to diffuse through the tissue fluid from capillary to cell. Waste products diffuse backwards from the cell into the tissue spaces back to the capillary. There are two mechanisms by which the body balances these fluids:

1. Diffusion: If a strong solution is separated by a membrane from a weaker solution, the substance dissolved, the solute, will pass from the strong solution to the weaker solution until the solutions have the same strength.

2. Osmosis: If a strong solution is separated by a membrane from a weaker solution but the membrane will not allow the solute to pass through, then water passes through in an opposite direction until both solutions have the same strength.

The capillaries behave as such a membrane with respect to the proteins in the plasma. The capillaries are permeable to water but impermeable to plasma proteins.

The biodynamic aspect of the tissue fluids

The biodynamic concepts embrace the totality of the activities and functions of the organism. In the micro-mechanisms of the alimentary tract, these principles take into account the physiological and emotional impacts and influences on the organism as well as taking into account the influence of the cosmic laws. Biodynamic principles explain the dimensions of the hormonal influences on the emotional reality of the organism and the basis of this study is to ask what is happening on all levels in the life of the organism, particularly in the central canal of the organism, the gut.

Orthodox study of the physiological mechanisms does not explain all the phenomena of the body fluids. At capillary level the tiny arteriole retains its smooth muscle coats until the capillary bed is reached. A circulating hormone, adrenalin for example, will only be absorbed if the vegetative cycle has been completed into full discharge and recuperation. The incompletion of the vegetative cycle[5] will result in minute traces of the hormone remaining in the muscle tissue where, later, biochemical changes take place. A minimal contraction in the arterial walls will result.

The two cosmic laws posited by Wilhelm Reich state that

1. Where there is a strong orgonotic field, water will be attracted to it.
2. Where there is a strong orgonotic field and a weak orgonotic field, the strong orgonotic field attracts energy from the weak field.

The strong orgonotic field at the capillary level will be contained in the arteriole walls. If a vegetative cycle has not been completed then the homeostatic fluid balance through osmosis and diffusion will be disturbed. If the situation becomes chronically unresolved, disturbed tissue will inevitably result. When this concept is orientated to the tissue of the gut an explanation for the presence of superfluous, unwelcome fluid in the walls of the gut is available. A chronic retention of the closure principle, as part of the vegetative cycle in the startle pattern, will cause chronic water logging in the intestinal tract walls.

Johannes Setekleiv throws further light on the workings of the intestinal tract. In his article, *The Spontaneous Rhythm Activity in Smooth Musculature*, Setekleiv[6] quotes the suggestion of the researcher Bozler[7] that there are two groups of smooth muscle:

---

5   Boyesen, Mona Lisa, 'Dynamics of the Vasomotoric Cycle', *Energy and Character*, Vol. 6, No. 2, 1975.

6   Setekleiv, Johannes, 'The Spontaneous Rhythm Activity in Smooth Musculature', published in *Tidskrift Norske Laegerforen,* 1964, from the Neuro-psychological Laborotory – Anatomical Institute, University of Oslo. Professor Med. Berger R. Kaadal. Translated from the Norwegian by Bente Schmid.

Multi-unit smooth muscle and
Single unit smooth muscle.

Bozler suggested that the multi-unit muscles are dependent for their contractile properties on a motoric nerve supply. Setekleiv says that one important feature of the single unit musculature is the stretch factor. He says:

> Reaction to passive stretching is an outstanding quality of bowel musculature. Quick-stretching triggers off a contraction – a stretch reaction. Further stretching decreases the ability of the musculature to have a stretch reaction.
> Over-stretching may occur from, for example, pathologically increased fluid in the pregnant uterus.

Bozler postulates that these single unit smooth muscle cells are found, for instance, in the intestinal tract, the ureters, the bladder and the uterus. Setekliev also says that the frequency of the spontaneous rhythmical contractions seems to be dependent on the length of the musculature.

The gut is almost ten convoluted meters in length. In general, these anatomical and physiological findings are the result of research on normal, healthy animal or human tissue. There was no focus in the research on the abnormalities of tissue disorganisation on the psychosomatic level. These findings, however, make the behaviour of pathologically fluid-filled gut walls more understandable. Still seeking to clarify the origins of lower back pain it is necessary to look at established scientific findings and the well tried phenomenological data. Episodic constipation alternating with diarrhoea and diagnosed as the condition, Irritable Bowel Syndrome, begs the question – what is the mechanism which triggers off the expulsion of the water from the walls to the lumen of the gut?

Homeostasis is as John Evans[8] says, 'an on-going, dynamic process that is only completely static in the absence of life'. The apparently abnormal behaviour of the colon in Irritable Bowel Syndrome is part of the

---

7   Bozler, E., 'Action Potentials and the Conduction of Excitation in Muscle'. *Biological Symposia 1941, 3, 95-109*, University of Oslo. Translated from the Norwegian by Bente Schmid.
8   Evans, John, *Mind Body and Electromagnetism*, Chapter 10, p.153, Element Books, 1986.

drive towards harmony on all levels. The whole of the intestinal tract is a complex and extraordinary organ. It is possible to live almost normally with no colon. Large portions of small intestine can be removed without disastrous consequences. If, however, it is handled roughly during surgical intervention, it can go into a life-threatening paralysis. It is a highly responsive organ.

The Body Electric

A factor that is crucial to life is the body's electrical system. Reich linked the cosmos to the way cosmic energy was transmuted or transformed into electricity as it approached the planet and found its way into all life. The minutest cell is an electrical organism. Any living animal or vegetable organism is an electrical system. Membrane potential and action potential infer the electric – the body electric. The electrical field surrounding each cell and system and finally the total organism is presently used in many therapeutic procedures in order to help promote the homeostasis and balance of life in the body. In the waterlogged gut the electrical system is disturbed by the abnormality of the tissues. The cell in its electrical field behaves abnormally. The pulsation is disturbed or even destroyed.

When organismic circumstances are moving towards pathology the organismic movement towards homeostasis persists. Wherever or whenever there is a living cell this momentum exists. According to biodynamic philosophy, levels of tissue disturbance include the physical manifestation of the unconscious (the Id) and the effects of the emotional on the individual. They are indivisible. The intestinal tract is the conduit for the Id. The communication mechanism of the central and peripheral nervous systems are the physical manifestations of the ego. The ego and the id can conflict with each other because we are human.

Psychoanalytic orientation

Synchronicity can sometimes change a whole perspective. I came across, quite by accident (!), an article in the *Journal of Psychoanalysis 1953* by

KR. Eissler, a colleague of Freud. He was writing about the emotionality of a schizophrenic patient. In 1938 Freud[9] had written that 'everything was at one time id. The ego was developed out of the continual influence of the outside world'. Eissler wrote

> At the beginning of development the id must have had free access to the perceptive apparatus which at that time was an apparatus receiving stimuli from the interior and discharging id energy.

As Freud hints in his hallucinatory wish fulfilment theory:

> The transformation of the perceptive apparatus into a nucleus of ego formation is probably one of the most decisive processes upon which the later fate of the ego will depend.

Although Eissler was not discussing a psychosomatic problem (or was it?) he continues

> One may construct the hypothetical model of an apparatus or of pathways along which excitations flow in opposite directions. The conclusion would be that these excitational flows must collide at one point.

It is not out of keeping with biological observations to assume, hypothetically, that such energies inhibit each other and lead to a formation of a structure. This mediating position of the perceptive apparatus, its biological faculty of the bearer of excitations flowing into opposing directions may make it the indispensable prerequisite for the formation of the ego nuclei.

My hypothesis is that this area of inhibition is the area of the ileo-caecal valve and the vermiform appendix.

The concept of the id canal, its vegetative nerve supply and, in part, its motoric central nervous system supply; led to the hypothesis that the human gut is constantly being subjected to up flows of the sympathetic nerve impulses. The organism has a deep need to counteract this when

9   Freud, Sigmund, 'The Ego and the Id – Anatomy of the Mental Personality', *New Introductory Lectures in Psycho Analysis*, 1932.

too much sympathetic activity creates imbalances. The para-sympathetic down flow supplies this need, most prominently in the gut.

Returning to our case history of Ann

Ann had a backache. Lower back pain was a recurring symptom. The relevance of this symptom came to my notice when I was told of the chiropractic theory of the great mimicker – the ileo-caecal valve area. This could be the structure, which, as Eissler postulated, could be the neutralising area for the conflict of the up and down flow of the energetic forces.

The ileo-caecal valve area includes the caecum with its appendix vermiformis. The area is well supplied by the protective lymph system and it has the ability to communicate to the organism that all is not well and to give the organism pain through the central nervous system. The chiropractic treatment of giving the open ileo-caecal valve a sharp shock impulse is to shock the valve, which is under too much pressure, into closing and stopping the abnormal fluid outflow. The valve normally opens and closes in response to the pressure of the contents of the lower ileum. The metabolic waste is passed rhythmically into the colon for disposal. The abnormal flow of fluid in diarrhoea disturbs the rhythm of the opening and closing valve.

The open valve, which responds to shock tactics, closes in a symp-tomatic relief. Bed-rest, sleep and relaxation adds to the organism's movement towards balance. Paying attention to the dietary intake can help this movement towards balance. The psycho-peristalsis is better able to resume its function when there is enough release of the fluid from the overloaded walls of the gut.

The situation for Ann was entirely resolved by a few treatments. Her lifestyle was a chronically damaging one. Physical and psychologi-cal help was needed and offered. The most valuable help would come from her own insights into why she continued to inflict over-stress on to her organism. Making a better relationship with her over stressed gut was a start.

The hypothesis of the link between the ileo-caecal valve syndrome and the lower back pain needs more thought, and more insights came from treating people with idiopathic lower back pain and tracing the histories backwards. The biological logic was there if it was possible to understand the mechanisms at work. The most important clinical revelation was that the lower back pain often began in very stressful periods of the patient's life. The reason for the stressful times were legion and human...family disruptions, divorce, examination time at school or college, too much driving vehicles under pressure, (taxi drivers, young ambitious business executives, media executives, and so on!).

Sometimes there was a grumbling appendix under medical supervision and ultimately surgery in order to remove the offending worm. Sometimes the back pain went away and sometimes it returned. Sometimes the pain moved up to the lumbar region and the lumbar-thoracic. In the beginning the pain had been lower down. Patient's histories revealed that, initially, the pain had often begun in the right sacroiliac joint. (viz. the chiropractors noted pseudo-sacroiliac strain) and later moved to the left sacroiliac joint.

The body seeks balance constantly. A contraction against pain, which can be very acute, in the right sacro-iliac joint can cause contraction in the right hip joint and the pelvis will tilt. In compensation, the left hip will try to adjust and take some of the strain. Pain across the lower back will result. So far, there has been a sequence of events beginning with an over stressed organism trying to live a normal life. As a result of the chemostatic fluid in the walls of the gut there has been in a chronic state an inability to discharge the excessive fluid because the gut walls are failing to act with a normal peristaltic movement. The walls of the gut become flaccid. The constant battle for homeostasis results in some of the fluid being discharged and diarrhoea results. The ileo-caecal valve behaves abnormally and can no longer hold back the flow of discharge. It resigns![10] The individual often finds that a period of constipation follows. However the gut has no chance to behave normally because the person persists in the over-stressful life style and the gut is then involved in the losing battle. The Irritable Bowel Syndrome is established.

Man is a social animal and not only the ego and the id are in conflict in the autonomic nervous system but there is also the other contender in

---

10   Too much chemostatic fluid between the muscular coats of the gut prevents normal pulsation. The peristaltic function of the gut becomes inhibited. It follows therefore that psycho-peristalsis will also be inhibited. The musculature becomes flaccid.

the battle for harmony. There is also the 'super-ego', which has a vocabulary of should and must. It is this contender which affects the over stressed organism just at the time when the organism is crying out for rest and attention. The area of gut at the ileo-caecal junction becomes less and less able to neutralise the conflict of the ego, the id and the super ego, until some pathology intervenes. The tissues of the terminal ileum and the caecum are affected by the chemostatic immobility. Stasis and immobility can be sustained for a time. The total gut is affected, however, and the pulsation so necessary for the health of tissue is disturbed. Psycho-peristalsis cannot digest the emotional hormonic remnants of the un-completed vegetative cycles. Stasis in tissue can affect a strong response from the immune system and the area of the caecum and appendix is well supplied with lymph tissue.

The omentum is an apron of protection by reason of its supply of lymph vessels, which responds to infection by moving to cover the area of infection. It is possible that the virus population in the tissue responds to the diminished life pulsation by becoming active in a milieu suited to it. In spite of the response of the lymph tissue and the efforts of the omentum (the apron of protection for the caecum and appendix), tissue is damaged by the viral activity and other pathogens join in. Maybe the vermiform appendix is meant to behave like an antenna to shake off the invaders. What is often observable is the increased amount of fluid in the abdomen at the time of surgical intervention for appendicitis.

Modern drugs and swift surgical intervention means that appendicitis is rarely life threatening. A less acute situation may occur and the immune system is more effective, active and efficient. The pain in the abdomen, fever and vomiting, as well as diarrhoea, settles down with, perhaps, the aid of an anti-biotic. The psycho-peristalsis, though not fully efficient, has benefited from the rest and the removal of fluid by the actions of the vomiting and diarrhoea. If the re-organisation of the all-important life style does not happen, the old pattern leading to the crisis situation will continue as soon as the crisis has passed.

The movement of energy to the periphery

The energy has centripetal directional movement towards the id canal in the early stages of the organism's response to the chronic over-stress. This may show itself in a period of depressive feelings. A critical situation such as a bout of pain accompanied by vomiting, fever, pain and tenderness settling in the right iliac fossa of the lower abdomen can follow the earlier depressive feelings. The energy has turned inwards towards the gut. When the crisis is over, the energy begins to move in a centrifugal direction. This is the life energy pattern of expansion ...moving towards the periphery.

The pelvic tensions, which have responded to the contractions in the thoracic diaphragm, have only partly been reduced and energy finds it difficult to permeate the static tissues. When energy encounters the tissue stasis it is likely that the plasma-faradic cleansing will only be an irritant to the nerve supply and pain in the right sacro-iliac joint will result. The joint, immediately behind the stressed ileo-caecal valve will be the first bony area to meet the energy.

Expansion meeting the sacro-iliac joint

This joint is slightly movable in the female, owing to the need to open the pelvis in the birth process. It is less movable in the male pelvis. As has been noted earlier, a resultant adjustment of the pelvic balance can produce evidence of strain in the left sacro-illiac joint. If the whole pelvic girdle is affected, the pain and stiffness can move upwards even as far up as the cervical spine. Sometimes the patient reports migraine-like headaches.

The sacro-illiac immobility can be compounded by an emotional response to the frustration of not being able to move freely and when this happens patients find difficulty in making a move to make a decision. There is an accompanying emotional response, a holding of the breath; a reduced diaphragmatic pulsation which reacts on the pulsation of the pelvic diaphragm and the psycho-orgastic pulsation.[11]

11   *Plasma-Faradic* is a concept that Gerda Boyesen applied to the cleansing action of life energy in tissue rendered static by chemostasis. See Glossary of Terms, p.152.

Over-stress as a way of life

Over-stress is not by any means the result of dramatic or tragic events in our lives. It is much more to do with the relentless impact of the small stresses. The small conflicts are what life is all about. Biodynamic philosophy says that the incompleted startle pattern is where much of our neuroticism begins. We are all victims of the process...if we choose to be victims.

Appropriate techniques in the treatment of idiopathic lower back pain

The techniques used in the treatment of idiopathic lower back pain can be varied and dependent on the physical state of the patient. For instance, a young child suffering from an anxiety state may not express the emotional pain as being in the lower back but may be responding to the over stress by pain in the belly and some vomiting. This situation, if there is a fever in the child, will always call for urgent medical attention since it is a potentially life threatening illness. If however the crisis settles, the fever and vomiting disappear but the reasons for the child's anxiety remain. In such a case, Energy Distribution treatment including some attention to the ileo-caecal valve will be very valuable as the child moves towards homeostasis. Some of the most effective biodynamic therapeutic treatments are

Energy Distribution Technique
Ileo-Caecal Valve Technique
Passive Lifting of the Shoulder Girdle tissues –- this helps towards making the breathing rhythms more free
Passive Jelly Fish Movements (to promote and encourage the life energy flow down through the pelvis towards a healthy grounding of the organism). The psycho-orgastic health of the organism depends on the free flow of life energy in the thoracic and pelvic structures.
Palming
Pulsatory Touch Technique
Palming and the Pulsatory Touch Technique are valuable in the treatment of the abdominal area. These gentle touch techniques are less likely to produce startle reactions in a vulnerable abdomen. At any time during a therapeutic session the patient may want to express in words or movements the feelings which are impinging from inside and all the space required for this should be allowed.

The Biodynamic Opening of the Shoulder Girdle

This technique involves giving a positive lifting and opening of the shoulder joints with a rhythm in tune with the patient's breathing. It is not to be confused with Bio-Release stretching and lifting.[12] Stretching should be kept to a minimum and only used after the lifting and only so that the limb may lie alongside the patient in as relaxed and natural position as possible.

Method of application

Stand facing the patient's right hand side as they lie supine on the massage table. Lift the patient's right limb by the wrist in as smooth a movement as possible. Don't fumble any more than you can help. A clean movement will avoid unnecessary startle patterns. With the right hand take the patient's right hand. In one movement stretch and extend the fingers of the patient's hand in tune with the patient's breath. Stretch on the in breath; relax on the out breath. Do this three times.

Still holding the patient's right wrist, stroke gently and firmly down the fingers to the fingertips and slightly beyond. Slide the left hand under the patient's left elbow and slightly above so that the patient's arm is held at a right angle. Lift the limb an inch or two with the patient's in breath until the patient's arm is above the head and slightly rotated outwards. If there is a reason, such as an arthritic condition, why these movements are restricted, stay with the restriction for one or two breath cycles when a spontaneous out breath may occur.

Now, begin to lower the limb with each out breath an inch or so at a time until the whole limb rests alongside the patient again. Use both hands to give a long firm but gentle stroke down the limb from shoulder to finger tips. Use this stroke three times. Move to the patient's left-hand side and repeat the technique with the therapist's left hand holding the patient's left hand and continuing the hand and finger stretching and shoulder lifting as before.

12   See Glossary of Terms

The Passive Jellyfish

Students who have studied and practised biodynamic psychotherapy will know that this method follows, but differs from the bio-release concept of the Jellyfish, adapted from Reich's important concept of Orgonomy.[13] A free flow of life energy through the pelvic structures has meaning on four levels, physical, emotional, energetic and etheric. A physically healthy pelvic area will present no restriction to the free flow of the circulating life energy.

No tissue in the organism is free from the risk of injury or even transitory disease. The ability to regain harmony is what health means. An emotional situation such as conflicting drives in opposite directions can result in going nowhere. 'I want to change my job. It's too badly paid and gives me no soul satisfaction. I can't do this because I have too many family responsibilities and I can't risk losing all the financial benefits of my present job. I'm stuck'.

This may be an uncomfortable situation but a physically healthy pelvis can move physically away and will use sport and exercise to be free for short periods. On the energetic level the organism's ability to maintain contact with its centre, its centre of gravity, its self, will be maintained and a well maintained awareness of this centre is reflected in its ability to stay grounded and to be able to face whatever life has to offer. This is balance on all levels of the life experience.

The Passive Jellyfish Technique

This technique is a lifting and stretching of the hip joints in tune with the patient's breath rhythm. The joints are moved one by one in the most sensitive way. The therapist is aware of the slightest resistance to the pelvic relaxation and under no circumstances will push through any such resistance. Instead the therapist stays with what is happening. The pelvic area can contain so much suppression and repression of expression that the amount of information stored there is enormous. It is the function of the biodynamic therapist to help the natural flow of energy to move through this area of powerful bones and muscles.

13   See Glossary of Terms

The use of the patient's breathing rhythms by the therapist is fundamental to this technique. When the thoracic diaphragm is fully connected to the pelvic hammock of structures there will be a full psycho-orgastic flow. When there is resistance to the opening of the hip joint the therapist will wait. It is a waiting with a communication. The biodynamic therapist knows about the time intervals of psycho-peristaltic response. Sometimes it is instantaneous, sometimes not. By staying with the place of resistance and observing the breath rhythms of the patient, the therapist can often find, at this point, the patient may go into deep relaxation or even sleep. The joint suddenly relaxes, there is a release breath and a burst of psycho-peristalsis; and the relaxed limb moves easily from or to the mid-line. This technique goes under the resistance. The giving in occurred in a deep alpha state. Sometimes, the patient, later on in the therapeutic session, may recall that they had had an image or a memory or a feeling.

Method

The patient is supine. The right leg is bent up into the jelly-fish position with flexed hip, flexed knee and with the therapist's hand resting firmly on the patient's instep to prevent the foot from sliding down the table. The therapist guides the patient's knee joint towards the patient's mid-line with the patient's in breath. The movement may only be an inch at a time. The initial intention is not to put any further startle patterns into the pelvic area. Then with a gentle pressure on the inner aspect of the knee joint the leg is guided away from the mid-line. Another in breath and the leg is guided away from the mid-line an inch at a time with the out breath.

As mentioned earlier, any resistance to further movement away from the mid-line must be treated sensitively. The areas between the legs should always be lightly draped; the vulnerability of this physical position for male and female should be cared for. The exposed sexuality can easily be the cause of some startle and much will depend on the sensitivity of the therapist. It will be obvious that any patient who has suffered any form of sexual abuse or in some cases surgical abortion would not be able to take this particular technique as part of their therapeutic programme, at least in the early stages of their therapeutic process.

It must always be remembered that very few damaged joints have absolutely no movement possible. Even a minute amount can be enormously beneficial to a rigid pelvis. The joint should be opened as much as the patient can tolerate. The limb is then straightened and allowed to rest on the couch at about fifteen degrees from the mid-line. The therapist will then repeat the technique on the other leg. The treatment should be completed by applying long flowing strokes from the hip area down to the toes.

The Ileo-Caecal Valve Technique

This technique is most effective when used as part of the Energy Distribution treatment. The tissues will then be prepared for a more free flow of energy. The Energy Distribution technique, as developed by Ebba Boyesen[14] remains the classical method of treatment for the encouragement of a down flow of energy needed for the counter influence of a chronic sympatheticatonia.

In addition to the classical method it is possible to add other release techniques which supplement the classical pattern of the Energy Distribution treatment. Many if not all, patients suffering from lower back pain have very light lung expansion. This is partly the result of chronic anxiety held into the thoracic diaphragm but there is also rigidity in the spine as a whole. As the patient lies on the table in a supine position the tensions in the lumbar curve result in a gap between the table surface and the lumbar curve. A release of the tensions in the thoracic muscles will often relieve discomfort in the length of the spine. This can result in a series of release breaths and an increase in the psycho-peristaltic activity.

Energy Distribution over the head and neck will entail mobilisation of all tissues of the skull, face and neck with the intention of mobilisation of life energy upwards from the head and downwards, which counteracts the directional Energy of the adrenalin flow. The junction of the

---

14   Boyesen, Ebba, 'The Essence of Energy Distribution', *Collected Papers of Biodynamic Psychology*, Volumes 1 and 2, Chapter 11, Biodynamic Psychology Publications, London, 1969-79.

cervical area with the base of the skull is vulnerable to painful rigidity. Time spent on the muscles supplying this area can produce relaxation and a lively psycho-peristaltic response.

Pain in the lower spine affects almost all the muscles from the occipitalis down to the gluteals, both superficial and deep. An effective touch therapy over the head and neck will notify the anatomical direction finders in the massage. The *sternocleidomastoid* muscle directs the hands down from the base of the skull to the insertion of the muscle at the clavicle end medially. An outward movement of the hands takes the intention of the massage outwards along the clavicle to the origin of the deltoid muscle then down the arm. All of these movements reduce the neurotic flexure patterns and open the shoulder joints for freer breathing patterns and a more efficient oxygenation of the tissues.

The Energy Distribution technique covers all layers of the body tissues, deep and superficial. In those patients with lower back pain, the front of the body can be distorted into a chronic flexure pattern. In working down the chest from the top of the sternum the contractions in the pectoral muscles, the underlying inter-costals and the attachments of these muscles to the sternum must all be attended to in therapy that includes touch. Lower down, the external oblique muscles, the *serratus anterior* and the *rectus abdominus* muscles are all involved in a fully free breathing pattern.

The touch strokes which are most effective in the Energy Distribution technique are when the strokes go downwards with the direction of the muscle fibres; or outwards from the mid-line. In mobilising the tissues of the back a very valuable additional technique is a rolling of the tissues down the spine. Using both hands gently but firmly lift the tissues from the underlying thoracic spine and move the tissue in a rolling movement down the spine to the lumbo-sacral junction. This movement of the tissues allows any chemostatic fluid in the muscle inter-spaces to be made available for absorption into the circulatory pattern. This rolling movement is called the Chinese Roll because it is used by the Chinese Barefoot Doctors as part of their massage repertoire.

Chemostatic fluid can be the cause of irritation to nerve endings. It is not the fluid which causes the pain but the chemostatic elements in the fluid. The rolling movements can be applied vertically or horizontally. The *teres* muscles are crucial to the most full breathing action and must be included in the massage technique. A firm stretching of the lumbar area will often produce deep release breaths. Continuing attention to the back brings into focus the left and right sacro-iliac joints.

As the patient is lying prone an alternative to a colonic massage can be applied. The therapist leans across the patient and with the left hand gently tucked under the lower costal area of the patient's thorax and with the right hand tucked gently under the right lower abdomen, a gentle pulling massage movement is begun. Using one hand after the other the whole of the patient's right abdominal area is treated. As the therapist's hand moves a little lower in the area the whole pelvic rim can be explored. This may often reveal some fibrositic nodules in the tissue along the pelvic rim and a gentle mobilisation of the tissue to change the blood supply direction and some emptying technique will often produce psychoperistaltic release sounds.

The sacro iliac joints may also reveal fibrositic nodules and these can benefit from some patient attention with firm mobilisation of the tissue. The *gluteal* muscles are very powerful and firm mobilisation will be needed. The direction of the treatment will be towards the periphery and down the middle of the upper thigh following the *semitendonosis* muscle which originates deep in the upper thigh at the iliac tuberosity. This is another good direction finder and leads the energy down the lower thigh towards the knee and the *gastrocnemeous* muscle, the tendon of Achilles, the heel and the rest of the foot.

The treatment of the right lower back is very important for the treatment of the ileo-caecal valve area. In very over stressed patients there may be no peristaltic activity to be heard. In this event it can be valuable to pay attention to the biofield over the area of the lower back, immediately above the ileo-caecal area. The therapist will be standing to the patient's left side. With one hand resting lightly on the patient's left shoulder, rest the right hand about an inch away from the patient and over the area above the ileo-caecal valve. Stay in this position until the palm of the hand responds to the patient's biofield. This may feel like a prickling or a pulsation and can be accompanied by some reluctant, hesitant sounds from the stethoscope. If the therapist lifts the right hand as though stretching something in the biofield more sounds may develop. A few moments spent on the bone, muscle and skin tissue followed by a continued change in the biofield can produce quite deep relaxation in the patient.

The therapist then moves to the right hand side of the patient. The abdominal massage to the patient's abdomen is repeated. The treatment to the left sacroiliac and the gluteals, the semitendonosis, the gastrocnemius, the tendon of Achilles and the rest of the foot is exactly as performed on the patient's right lower back. Long strokes from the cervical region down to the tips of the toes. The patient then turns into the supine position. They are often surprised to find that they feel much more comfortable than at the beginning of the treatment session and the feeling of relaxation is very welcome. As the patient is lying in the supine position, bending the knees can relieve residual tension in the back muscles. The knees can touch but the feet should be about nine inches apart.

The Ileo Caecal Valve contact

The therapist lays his/her right hand over the area of the ileo-caecal valve which is about the centre of a triangle, the three points of which are the tip of the crest of the ilium, the umbilicus, and the tip of the pubic bone. It is McBurney's point mentioned in the medical diagnosis of acute appendicitis. A very gentle palpation of the deep tissue in this area may reveal some tenderness, but not an acute pain. Very gentle circular movements over the area can produce some psychoperistaltic sounds.

The therapist's left hand, meanwhile is under the patient's right lower back. A gentle Pulsatory Touch between the therapist's hands can be valuable. Gentle pressure is given as the two hands move towards each other with the patient's in-breath and release as the patient breathes out. This touch can be maintained for two or three minutes. Long strokes from head to toe are now applied to the whole of the left-hand side of the patient.

The patient then turns over on to the left side with the knees drawn up. The therapist can continue stimulating the lower back energy field. The area of the ileo-caecal valve can be held between the therapist's left hand, which is placed over the front aspect of the ileo-caecal valve area, and the right hand which is placed over the patient's lower back at the right hand side. The therapist continues the Pulsatory Touch for two or more minutes and then can use more stimulation of the biofield in this area. Long strokes down the patient's back completes the treatment from head to toes.

A last touch to the patient's head is always welcome. The protective blanket covering the patient protects them from the results of startle reflex patterns produced by their exposure to unfamiliar touch therapies.

In conclusion

In order that the therapist can pay the fullest attention to the needs of the patient, there should be as much information available as possible. This can be difficult to do when there is a limited amount of time available for an interview. The patient may omit very relevant information because they simply forgot or because they felt it was not relevant to their treatment or even the condition for which they are currently seeking help. Certainly there will be huge gaps in the initial picture.

There will, however, be enough for the therapist to begin to see the thread of the biologic and throughout the treatments there will be additions made to the case history. Any chronic illness is accompanied by a great weariness. The ill body is a weary body and is matched by a great weariness of the psyche. There is forgetfulness.

Depression comes with an overload of exhausting thoughts, which go round and round with no end to the exhaustion in sight and there is too little good quality sleep. Appetite for life is very poor. Sensuality is at a low ebb. Irritability and explosive behaviour are out of proportion to the irritating event. There can be withdrawal and a disinclination to talk about how they feel...they may not be able to feel.

All of these symptoms are in the body, the soma. In the use of the word psychosomatic there is an implication and recognition that the psyche and the soma are inextricably linked. The term psychogenic implies that the origin of the somatic disorder comes from psychological conflict or, at least, some psychological disturbance and imbalance.

It often appears from the patient's medical and social history that the healthy communication and harmonious interplay breaks down and the soma in many psychosomatic conditions appears to take on the job of attempting to harmonise and balance the conflicts on the road to homeostasis.

The idiopathic lower back pain can shelter many stories of pain and hurt deep in the psyche. Sometimes the soma is unable to find a way back to the psyche and there is only chronic somatic pain. Under these circumstances it is necessary to treat the presenting symptom or pain (that which is closest to the ego.)

Experience demonstrates how the result of attending to the chronic somatic pain uncovers the psychological dimension in a most genuine way; and re-establishes the essential link between psyche and soma. This is the true value of the application of biodynamic theories, concepts, principles and techniques.

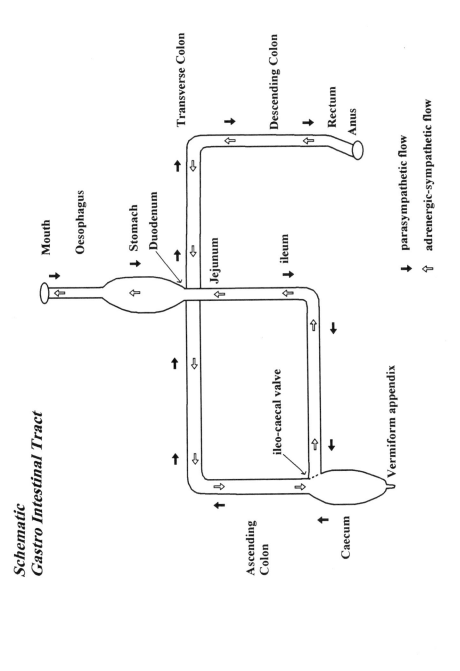

Schematic
Gastro Intestinal Tract

Mouth

Oesophagus

Stomach
Duodenum

Jejunum

ileum

Transverse Colon

Descending Colon

Rectum
Anus

ileo-caecal valve

Vermiform appendix

Ascending
Colon

Caecum

→ parasympathetic flow

⇨ adrenergic-sympathetic flow

CHAPTER 5

The broken coccyx, the kundalini and the psycho-peristalsis.

Theory and hypothesis begin with the experience of a cognitive insight. They are the result of a series of experiences that fit together within a phenomenological framework. When a jigsaw puzzle is put together, the picture on the box lid gives an overall idea of what the finished puzzle will look like. However, the picture is only a little representation of a particular item or view or picture.

There is an infinite extension beyond the puzzle and this is the problem with an hypothesis that has an anecdotal quality. The anecdote, however, must include some basic truths and in this chapter the anecdotal histories are of this nature.

The reason for this chapter begins with a gathering of dancers, aerobic practitioners and teachers. This group was to be addressed from the rostrum by three distinguished physicians who came to communicate their approvals and their anxieties. One of the physicians was the late Dr. Chandra Sharma,[1] who had a breadth of vision relating to the human condition. He said,

> When teaching people to exercise their bodies either gently or boisterously, we must remember the intricacies of our four circulatory systems. These are the arterial system, the venous system, the lymphatic system and the cerebrospinal fluid system.

I had not considered the latter system in the context of why we were altogether in this venue. However, the significance of the cerebrospinal fluid circulation became an important factor, later on, in my practical therapeutic experience.

A short time later, Mrs K. was referred to me by one of these physicians for therapy to help her to relax. She was a married lady, 44 years old. While on holiday abroad she had been shopping in the nearby city.

---

1   Sharma, Chandra, Unpublished Lecture

She experienced a sudden and severe chest pain. She was rushed to hospital and admitted into the intensive care unit of the cardiology department.

When the necessary tests and treatment had been given, the cardiologist told her that there was no sign of her having had a heart attack. Her heart was good for her age he said, but he advised her to consult a cardiologist on her return to England. This she did. The London cardiologist confirmed that there was no sign of heart disease but because of the shock of the experience and the patient's lingering anxiety about her health, a course of biodynamic treatment was advised.

Mrs K. was married to a restaurateur. The business was a busy one and Mrs K. and her husband worked together. The hours of work were long but she enjoyed it. At the interview, she told me that what she needed now was a feeling of reassurance that she was not a 'heart' patient.

The first treatment session

When the initial introduction and interview were completed, I outlined the therapeutic technique I would use that day. Since the physician had told her that she would be having massage, I outlined the Energy Distribution technique. This treatment would go some way towards helping in the reduction of the residual stress factors that continued to trouble Mrs K. She had not yet ever had any physiotherapy treatment.

She felt tensions in many parts of her body. She felt that an overall massage was what she needed although she had never experienced one. We made an initial contract for six sessions with a week between each session and the situation could be reviewed after the fourth treatment session. Treatment was needed to counteract the muscular tensions in her body. She had suffered a shock, and the anxiety of wondering whether she had had a heart attack remained with her, despite reassurance to the contrary.

The most appropriate massage technique to use in the circumstances was Energy Distribution. This massage counteracts the effects of shock. Shock produces stasis that continues to feed anxiety feelings. Energy Distribution is an overall massage with a downward direction. The anxiety hormones, such as adrenalin, have an upward directional flow. This massage produces a calming effect through the production of the hormones that counteract the upward flow of the anxiety hormones and bring relaxation to the body. The treatment lasts for 50 minutes.

At the beginning of the treatment Mrs K. had painfully contracted muscles in her face and neck. She breathed in a shallow manner because of the tensions in her diaphragm. She enjoyed the massage and though the sounds from the stethoscope were intermittent, there were responsive watery sounds from the psycho-peristalsis, which followed any spontaneous breath Mrs K. released. When Mrs K. turned over on to her left side at the end of the treatment there were more continuous sounds. Mrs K. had been able to digest the old stress products and this was an indication of her underlying positive health. The muscles of her face were softer and her skin was pinker. Mrs K. rested for ten minutes.

The second treatment session

One week later, Mrs K. said she had felt lighter when she left after the last treatment session. This feeling lasted for a few days. Mrs K. was given a further Energy Distribution massage during the second treatment. She relaxed more easily and quickly. I heard some loud psycho-peristaltic sounds as I was treating the areas round the eyes and the base of the skull. A resting pressure touch was used over these areas when these sounds came from the stethoscope and the pressure was maintained until the sounds lessened in volume. The treatment lasted for fifty minutes and Mrs K. rested for ten minutes before leaving.

The third treatment session

One week later, Mrs K. had nothing to say about the last treatment session. She smiled and said that she was looking forward to the treatment. I began the third Energy Distribution massage. The psycho-peristaltic sounds came more immediately when I massaged the muscles over the skull, the muscles of the face and behind the ears in the mastoid process area. This produced continuous mixed watery and electric sounds. The less tense Mrs K. became the more continuous release sounds fitted into the picture of an undoing of the overstress pattern.

As she lay supine on the table, biodynamic massage to her hands and feet produced more continuous sounds than before. The sounds were less explosive and there were occasional little bursts of watery sounds. Mrs K. was releasing the old static hormonal remnants, which had been causing pain in her neck muscles. The release sounds from her hands and feet indicated a progressive release of tensions going down her body and reflected the validity of the concept behind the massage. Mrs K.'s once painful places were now less painful or pain-free. Mrs K.'s breathing was more full, indicating a lessening of tension in her diaphragm. It was possible to see or feel the areas where changes were taking place. I brought this to her attention.

As she lay prone for the second half of the treatment, I continued to loosen the muscles of the back over the diaphragm. The Energy Distribution technique includes assisting the movement of energy round the connective tissue and the muscle covering tissue. I lifted the tissue away from the ribcage. As I did so there was an increase in the volume of the psycho-peristaltic sounds. The shock of the painful heart experience had produced contractions in the *trapezius* on both sides of her neck. The muscles of the lower thoracic area, the *latissimus dorsi* and the *teres minor and major* muscles had all contracted with the experience of the pain. They had not fully relaxed when the pain had receded.

The spaces between the muscles were affected by the retention of the old hormone remnants that are the result of the emotion of fear in the undischarged startle. This build up of tension and the attracted fluid makes chemostasis. Touch and the mobilisation of the tissues produce more psychoperistaltic sounds and these were louder and more continuous than before. Working with the tissue in this way is very valuable but time consuming and time is not limitless. It is necessary that the therapist is aware of the importance of the emergence of emotional expression. This indicates a completion of an old uncompleted cycle. The therapist must allow time for this emotional expression, and for it to be worked through. Mrs. K. was experiencing the completion through an active psycho-peristalsis. The undoing of old tensions was proceeding.

Long effleurage strokes from the top of the spine down through the body were applied. From the lower thoracic region down through the lumbo-sacral and through the middle of the sacrum surface, the sounds were intermittently explosive then loud and continuous. This indicated that there had been a build up of tensions down the whole of the spine. It seems that these tensions had been relieved by the touch of the effleurage strokes.

When the sacrum and coccyx were reached the sounds were intermittently explosive, then loud and continuous. The spinal column area had produced sounds through the psycho-peristalsis as though it were a musical instrument with a variety of decibels. The curve of the sacrum continued into the curve of the coccyx. The gluteal cleft produced very loud and explosive sounds. I traced the coccygeal curve to the point where it came to an abrupt angle. This was a more precise palpation than effleurage strokes. This angularity was abnormal and felt like an old fracture. The sounds along the coccygeal periosteum were very loud and explosive.

Contact with the periosteum of the coccyx was continued until the tip of the coccyx was reached. There was no pain as the touch was maintained at the tip of the coccyx. After a minute or so the quality of the sounds changed. The loud explosive sounds diminished and watery sounds were interspersed with no sound. This period of treatment lasted about 15 minutes. The more gentle sounds and Mrs. K's obvious relaxation indicated a change in the energetic situation. Nothing in Mrs. K's medical history revealed that she had a history of damage to her lower spine. To explore this lack of information at this point in the therapy would disturb her relaxation and so it was left until the next session one week later.

The fourth treatment session

Mrs. K was very excited when she arrived for the weekly treatment. Since the last session she had found herself taking many more deep breaths than usual. Three days after her treatment she was having supper with her family when suddenly her nose began to stream clear fluid. She had no fever and no sign of a cold. She left the supper table and for some hours she experienced this flow of clear fluid from her nose. She said, I used a whole box of tissues. The following day she felt very tired and drained. Now, she talked excitedly about this flowing response to the treatment and said that nothing like this had ever happened to her before.

I treated her with the Energy Distribution massage because it was effective but also to explore any changes. The psycho-peristaltic sounds were less explosive throughout the treatment and the liquid sounds came readily, particularly over her face and, when she lay prone, over her thoracic diaphragm. When the massage reached the sacrum and the beginning of the coccygeal curve there was a clear reduction in the volume of the explosive sounds. I explored the periosteal response at the tip of the coccyx and the sounds were continuous with more of the liquid sounds than in the last session. Together with Mrs. K's buoyant mood there was reason to think that the change in the psycho-peristaltic sounds indicated relief in the amount of chemostasis reduction.

So far, in this session, I had not probed into the history of the deformity in the coccyx. The curve of the coccyx changing into an angle did indicate possible damage but further information was so far not forthcoming. Mrs. K. was so comfortable with herself that it was not necessary to probe. Had she shown anxiety or any other symptom requiring more of a psychotherapeutic approach that would have been a different situation. The coccyx area is fraught with potential problems. Sensitivity and a good rapport with the patient help to keep the problems to a minimum.

There was no hint in the medical history that Mrs. K. had any psychosexual problems and her relaxed response to last week's treatment was encouraging. Nevertheless it was important to be very sensitive in this lower pelvic area. The coccyx, when naturally curved, leads the energy flow over the perineum and up the front of the body. The health of the perineum and inner and outer vaginal tissue is very important for a woman's healthy sexuality. A good balance of all the energy input is crucial and this includes the vegetative system. The treatments so far were meant, through the Energy Distribution technique, to encourage a balance and this meant a parasympathetic response to counteract the chronic sympatheticotonia. The present treatment was in accordance with this principle. Mrs. K. enjoyed the relaxation that was the response to the massage.

There was also a significant factor emerging. She said she felt relaxed when she thought about having a treatment. There was a significant conditioning element. The fourth session had, now, come and gone. Mrs. K. confirmed her commitment to further treatment and I suggested that we made a contract for a further four treatments. She agreed.

The fifth treatment session

We began by Mrs. K. telling me that the Cardiology consultant had seen her. He had declared her free of cardiac pathology. I had in the meantime spoken to this doctor and told him about my theory of Mrs. K. having at some time, damaged her coccyx. He thought that this was in no way relevant to a cardiac pain. I asked her, now, whether she had at any time hurt herself.

She immediately remembered an episode when she was eight years old. She had fallen down cellar steps in her home. Her father was dead and she was required to help her mother in the little teashop they had. She also had to help with two younger siblings. On this occasion she wanted to go out to play but her mother needed something from the cellar. The resentful little girl had to do this before she was allowed out. She remembers falling down the steps and landing on her bottom on the stone step. Her mother was angry and the little girl got no sympathy for having hurt herself and having a painful tail. During the telling of this event Mrs. K. showed no emotion or any surprise that in the intervening years she had never recalled the event.

The treatment for this session was the Energy Distribution massage. When the coccyx was reached, the touch over the coccyx produced less explosive sounds. There was no pain. Mrs. K. said she was able to breathe more deeply and said, 'I feel as though I'm breathing properly for the first time in my life'. Together with this and partly as a result of it, she said she could smell things more acutely. During the next few weeks, she began to feel very alive and well. She said she realised that she had never felt well; that she had always been 'marginally depressed'.

After this period of treatment she experienced a well being which was a totally new experience for her. The consultant from whom she had been referred considered her to be cured after six treatment sessions and no longer in need of therapy for relaxation. There was no medical comment on a possible link between the dramatic chest pain and the old fracture of the coccyx. The patient thought otherwise.

An Australian psychiatrist friend told me that she habitually asks her patients during their initial interview whether they had sustained damage to the lower spine. She suggested that I read Dr. Lee Sanella's book *The Kundalini Experience*.[2] The question to be answered was: Was there a connection between the sudden chest pain when Mrs. K. was in her middle years and the fall down the cellar steps when she was eight years old?

An energetic review of the events

Mrs. K. experienced her chest pain while she was on holiday in the warmth of South America. She was unwinding with friends. Her over-stress levels would be reduced in this atmosphere by the unimpeded self-regulatory mechanisms. The safe, secure atmosphere encouraged her relaxation. Ever since the traumatic event 36 years ago, the young, hurt, 8-year old child lingered in a memory, which appeared to have been locked into the broken tissue of her coccyx area. She remembered that she hadn't cried much. She said, 'I put up with the pain until it went away'.

Her self-regulation, her ability to move towards harmony and homeostasis continued to function quite well over the years so the dramatic event during her holiday was a mystery. She had given birth to two children without problems and she maintained a good level of health in the intervening years. She could recall no details of how the pain behaved, whether it was a static pain or whether it moved in any direction.

Having read Dr. Sanella's book *The Kundalini Experience* and found no reference or case history concerned with a fractured coccyx, I nevertheless found the following passage which was interesting and could be relevant.

> In the course of its upward motion, the kundalini is held to encounter all kinds of impurities that are burned off by its dynamic activity. In particular, the Sanskrit scriptures mention three structural blockages, which are known as knots.

2   Sanella, Lee, *The Kundalini Experience – Psychosis or Transcendence*, Integral Publishing, California, 1987.

According to traditional understanding, these knots are located at the lowest centre in the anal area, the heart centre and the centre between and behind the eyebrows...but the pathway of the kundalini can be blocked anywhere along its trajectory.

We can look upon these blockages as stress points. Thus in its ascent, the kundalini causes the central nervous system to throw off stress. This is usually associated with pain.[3]

So says Dr. Sanella in the chapter on the Physio-Kundalini in his book *The Kundalini Experience – Psychosis or Transcendence*. Medical orthodoxy recognises nothing comparable to the kundalini. It would be breaking new ground if a connection were formulated that considered taking the kundalini, the psyche and the soma as the conceptual view of Mrs. K.'s heart pain. So far I have failed to find anything in the literature which connects fractures of the coccyx with somatic disease following in due course.

The Kundalini Energy

In the Yogic tradition the kundalini energy is situated in the base of the spine. The coccyx, in the yogic tradition is the root centre. Here, the energy has reached its lowest rate of vibration. In relation to sound this would be something approaching the deepest note of the tuba or the double bassoon. I had noted early in my treatment of Mrs K.'s spine, that sounds of the psycho-peristalsis resembled the decibels of the sound of a musical instrument. These psycho-peristaltic sounds changed noticeably, as I worked down the spine to the coccyx area.

In Hindu terminology, this vibration is called a Tattwa and in Western esoteric terms as an element. The element of the root chakra has the quality of solidity. It is the earth element. When stimulated there can be a noticeable urge for the individual to move the feet by marching or dancing. Traditionally, the Earth Element gives the quality of resistance and solidity against gravity. A good Earth Element gives a feeling of having one's feet on the ground and the sense of being able to smell the earth. The sense of smell is very important to the earthed individual. Mrs. K.

3   Sanella, Lee, *The Kundalini Experience – Psychosis or Transcendence*, Integral Publishing, California, 1987.

had remarked on the improvement in her sense of smell after the fifth week of treatment.

Eastern tradition says that the Energy Centre above the root chakra is the sacral centre at the level of the sacrum. This element is of water and the experience of this centre is one of fluidity in the inner being. With the sacral centre we experience a fullness, a ripeness and this element is when a human being is ripe for full sexuality. This fluidity gives the experience of flow. This fluidity is also contained in the movement of the snake. The old tradition relates the movement of the kundalini energy to the coiled up snake in the sacral chakra ready to rise up through the spine towards the supreme centre in the brain. This energy washes the tissues before descending from its peak. Fluid and the washing mechanisms of the kundalini energy have a physiological manifestation. This is the cerebro-spinal fluid (CSF).

The Central Nervous System

The central nervous system is the communication system between the individual organism and the Environment. It includes the brain and spinal chord. Three membranes cover the brain, externally: the *Dura Mater* – the outer layer, the *Arachnoid Membrane* – the middle layer and the *Pia Mater* – the inner layer which is adherent to the brain.

The cerebro-spinal fluid (CSF), which resembles lymph, surrounds the brain in the sub-arachnoid space between the arachnoid and the pia mater, and fills the space ventricles within the brain. The four principle ventricles are the right and left lateral ventricles, one in each cerebral hemisphere; the third ventricle, which communicates by the inter ventricular foramina and the fourth ventricle which lies in the medulla. This ventricle communicates with the spinal canal of the spinal cord. This is a minute canal.

The Spinal Cord

The Spinal Cord is about 17 inches (43 cm.) long and is about 0.5 inches (1.3 cm.) in diameter. It lies in the vertebral canal and extends from the medulla to the level of the 2nd lumbar or between the 1st and 2nd lumbar vertebrae.

The Peripheral Nervous System

There are twelve pairs of cranial nerves arising from the brain. In addition there are 31 pairs of spinal nerves arising from the spinal cord. The whole of the nervous system, the central nervous system and the peripheral nervous system, are intimately connected with the cerebro-spinal fluid. Although the spinal cord terminates between the 1st and 2nd lumbar vertebrae, there is a continuation of the cerebro-spinal fluid flow down to the lumbar theca. This is the space extending beyond the end of the spinal cord and into the sacrum.

The Cerebro-Spinal Fluid Circulation

This fluid is formed from vascular secretion lining the ventricles of the brain. It circulates within the folds of the brain and the spinal cord and is in constant movement where life exists. It covers the brain and acts as a buffer of protection. It provides nutrition and a means of removing metabolic waste through the venous sinuses. There is a continuous circulation of this fluid from the blood vessels in the ventricles throughout the central nervous system. Then it is re-absorbed into the venous circulation ready for the next secretory flow from the ventricles of the brain.

In general the CSF is only brought to the attention of the man in the street if it is necessary to remove some of it by lumbar puncture. It is then sent to the laboratory for examination in order to discover the identity of the germ or other pathological organism suspected of causing damage or disease in the central nervous system. It is, of course, known that the central nervous system tissues are moistened by a fluid, but the importance of this extraordinary fluid is given scant attention other than its importance as a physiological factor in the central nervous system.

Professor W.E. Le Gros Clark in his textbook *The Tissues of the Body*[4] gives the following information, the only mention made of the cerebro-spinal fluid. It has been shown, however, that there are reciprocal volume changes between the blood and the cerebro-spinal fluid varying in magnitude with the position of the body.

Gross anatomy and physiology in the period before the Second World War and up to the present time does not include any hints of the more subtle functions of the CSF. Sir W.E. Le Gros Clark quotes L.H. Weed in the article on the Meninges and Cerebro-Spinal Fluid.[5] Weed suggests that

> The chief function of the CSF may be to allow a prompt reciprocal adjustment in response to changes that occur in the amount of blood in the arteries and veins within the skull.
> Certainly, any rise in arterial or cerebro-spinal fluid pressure will tend to obstruct the venous flow from the brain.

Recent literature on the gross anatomy and physiology of the central nervous system shows no hint of more subtle functions of the CSF. Such information could throw light on the connection, if any, between a fractured coccyx and a severe heart pain with no demonstrable pathology, thirty years after the fracture was sustained.

I recalled reading an article expounding a theory, which could explain, in part, how the sap of a tree rises up through the trunk. The theory postulated that the canopy of branches and twigs and leafage as spring began, produced a strong energy field that would, in accordance with Reichian Laws, act with a hydrative effect. The fluid sap would be attracted to the strong energetic and electro-magnetic field of the canopy and hence rise.

In the human being, the strong and powerfully energetic brain at the top of the spinal column could also behave as the tree behaved. The cerebro-spinal fluid rising towards the strong field. In its early development the human baby has a proportionately larger head than an adult and has a greater intellectual potential. Physiological and biological sciences do not, yet, fully explain the total function of the CSF.

---

4   Le Gros Clark, W.E., *The Tissues of the Body*, Chapter 13, (p. 413), Oxford University Press, 1975.
5   Weed, L.H., 'Meninges and Spinal Fluid', *Journal of Anatomy*, 72, 1938.

Theories based on rhythmic, physical pulsations in the body as a whole together with new findings relating to electro-magnetic influences and the subtle sub-molecular and sub-atomic influences, still have to be brought together and synthesised with all modern physiological findings.

As neuro-physiology finds out more, and researchers find out more, the prospects of finding more answers to the questions relating to organic behaviour become more and more exciting. Some will confirm previously held dogma and some will be refuted. What does seem clear, however, is that the CSF has function and movement. The understanding of this function and movement is gradually unfolding.

The rising and raising of the kundalini

In the Yogic tradition, the kundalini rises from the base of the spine in a natural progression. It can also be raised in a contrived and manipulated technique using meditation and breath. In the standing yogic meditation there is a deliberate moving upwards of the kundalini energy by producing standing vibrations in the body and bringing the influence of the breath into the upwards direction.

In life, the kundalini energy is constantly on the move. The phenomenon is natural and necessary to the organism in order that healthy functioning should be maintained throughout the body. Similarly, the phenomenon of the psycho-peristalsis is a natural and necessary healing body mechanism. Both the kundalini and the psycho-peristalsis are tuned to the natural contraction and expansion, the pulsation, of all living tissue.

The movement of the kundalini energy is upwards towards the nerve centre of the brain but it also returns to the place from whence it came, the base of the spine. It affects the whole of the organism through the nervous systems, the central, peripheral and the vegetative nervous systems. If injury or disease strikes the organism the balancing functions of the kundalini and the psycho-peristalsis will be needed and they have to be in maximum health.

In the raising of the kundalini in the Yogic meditation, strong stress patterns are used in using the body as a vibrational organism. As a result a wave is produced in the spinal movement. This is what Ebba Boyesen calls the orgastic wave.[6] There is an involvement of the breath and, there-fore, the diaphragm. The full potential for healthy pulsation in the dia-phragm will depend on the physical and emotional health of the organ-ism.

The kundalini meditation can affect the psyche and produce dra-matic changes in the organism. Breath is the key factor in these changes. Vibrational movement will not in itself produce raising of the kundalini. Breathing is the necessary function that keeps the organism alive. No breath...no life.

Case History 1

P.J., a forty-year old male, took part in a standing kundalini meditation based on the psycho-orgastic vibrations as described by Ebba Boyesen.[7] The exercise was performed to music with an alpha beat and lasted over one and a half hours. P.J. intended to drive away at the end of the exer-cise and make a journey of some forty miles.

At the end of the exercise his breathing was shallow but not unduly fast. His ability to focus attention in the here and now was impaired and from time to time he shook from head to foot with wave-like vibrations. After resting for an hour and having several cups of black coffee, P.J. appeared to have his balance on all levels restored. He knew where he was and who he was and there was no further shaking. He knew what he intended to do and felt competent to drive to his destination and back. His breathing was deeper and he appeared to be well grounded and to-tally coherent. His companion sat with him as he drove for the next hour. The companion kept up a conversation and encouraged P.J. to maintain an awareness of his breathing patterns and on the here and now.

P.J. appeared to be normal when the destination was reached. They had a sandwich and a cup of coffee in a restaurant and then, the compan-ion saw that P.J's concentration was slipping and vibrations throughout his body were re-occurring. P.J. was put to rest on his left side and he

6   Boyesen, Ebba, 'The Psycho-Orgastic Vibration', *Energy and Character*, Abbots-bury Publications, 1978, and *Collected Papers of Biodynamic Psychology*, Vol-umes 1 and 2, Biodynamic Psychology Publications, London. 1979.
7   *Ibid.*

slept for an hour. At the end of this time he woke up and was back in the here and now, fully, with no apparent ill effects. After this he drove a further 40 miles and then slept, non-stop, for over 12 hours.

Many questions need answers as a result of P.J.'s experience.

Case History 2

A television programme showed a Tibetan healer in his country preparing to treat a lady suffering from migraine. He was accompanied by an acolyte. The television camera showed the healer preparing himself for the healing session by using a deep breathing technique. The healer stood upright while the acolyte stood near in attendance. The healer began to take deep, deep breaths while the commentator explained that the healer was directing his breath down to the base of his spine.

After some minutes the healer began to vibrate from, head to foot. The acolyte meantime, supported the healer while the shaking continued. The migraine sufferer was, in the meantime, sitting and smoking a cigarette looking very composed and tranquil. She gave no sign of suffering any kind of pain. This is common in Western treatment for migraine. Patients will commonly seek help for their migraine pain between attacks.

The Tibetan healer at no time touched his patient but while being supported by the acolyte he began to pull handfuls of an unseen something from the lady's head and then from the rest of her body as she sat smoking her cigarettes. At no time did anyone speak and after some minutes of the ritual she got up and walked away. We viewers were not told of any subsequent healing.

The word kundalini was not mentioned but migraine pain and the ritual were understandable in this demonstration. It was also a demonstration that migraine is not confined to the over-stressed Western population.

The Yogic manipulation of the life force, particularly in Hatha Yoga, is known as pranayama often translated as breath control. Most, if not all, meditative techniques have some kind of breath control as part of their discipline; and some authorities warn against the injudicious and uninformed use of pranayama as a means of accelerating the ascent of the kundalini energy. Dr. Lee Sanella[8] warns

> Deliberate practice of these methods by forcing the kundalini, may cause premature and imbalanced release of titanic forces.

An upright stance is not necessary for the upward movement of the kundalini force. Many people, as Dr. Sanella reports, experience the symptoms that accompany the raising of the kundalini while they are lying down. The majority of those people who experience dramatic kundalini events have practised meditation of one kind or another or have been involved in prayer meditation or have taken psychedelic substances.

The accompanying breathing, the concentration and the resulting relaxation are not to be compared with the natural and gentle flow of the kundalini, which rises and falls and permeates all tissues with its effect, in an unconscious flowing movement. This is the way of the psychoperistalsis. In life it happens as a continuum. When there is an impediment in its progress towards harmony the organism will show signs of disorder or disturbance. There is then a need for therapeutic intervention.

Psycho-Peristalsis and the Kundalini

Dr. Sharma highlighted the blood circulation system and also the cerebro-spinal fluid circulation in his address to the dance practitioners. All the organismic systems are interwoven in his attention to the body under stress and this includes the esoteric aspects of the systems.

The Respiratory System

Life can only be maintained if the organism has the pulsatory ability to exchange nutrients and waste products at the basic cell level and the peripheral level. The inner environment communicates with the outer. The respiratory system is the oxygen provider for this. This is the

---

8   Sanella, Lee, *The Kundalini Experience – Psychosis or Transcendence*, Integral Publishing, California, 1987.

physiological function of the respiratory system. The esoteric breath of life is an ancient concept but it is as powerful and poignant today as it ever was. It has an emotional and spiritual dimension that is profoundly human.

The Digestive System

This system includes the intestinal tract for nutritional metabolism and is closely interwoven with the physiological respiratory system. The intestinal tract is easily reduced to having disorders if the oxygenation is impaired. This central tube has inherited its primitive origins from the worm. It has retained its worm-like movements in the digestive peristaltic action. The epithelial lining has developed from the endoderm germ layer. Its embryonic development results in the most inner layer of cell being, at least phenomenologically, the transporter of the most primitive impulses.

This is the 'id canal' as conceived by Gerda Boyesen when she described the gut as being the id canal; the conduit for the instinctive drives. Its secondary function is to digest the emotional waste products so that the healthy pulsation of all the tissues is maintained. This Gerda Boyesen named the 'psycho-peristalsis'. We show our awareness of this vulnerable central tube when we say:

> I have a gut feeling
> He's a worry guts
> He is gutless
> He is gutsy
> He is full of guts
> He makes me sick...and so on.

The Blood Circulation System and the Heart

This system is for pumping and transporting oxygen to all the body tissues. The heart muscle is an amazing structure that can work efficiently for a hundred years without stopping. The esoteric concept is in all languages:

My heart is full
My heart is heavy
From the bottom of my heart
My heart is breaking
My heart aches...and so on.

The cerebro-spinal fluid circulation pattern

The physical cerebro-spinal fluid has already been described and it too has an esoteric aspect to it. We have little in our Western idiom or vernacular that uses the esoteric perception of the cerebro-spinal fluid. There may be some relevance in the way we use the word 'high' when we feel transported by the beauty of a scene or a wonderful musical experience. The user of psychedelic drugs can feel on a 'high'.

Esoteric concepts come from the ancient Eastern wisdoms and languages. The acceptance of the ecstatic experiences and psychic changes of the Dervish dancers and African tribal dancers is not normally matched in the western world. The word kundalini is from the Sanskrit, meaning 'she who is coiled', and this has little to compare with anything in Western tradition or orthodoxy.

The concept of kundalini – 'she who is coiled' however echoes the concept of the energy flowing through the coiled gut in Gerda Boyesen's id canal. The spinal canal and the gastro-intestinal canal are both conduits for the flow of energy. The common circulatory system that unites the total organism is the heart and blood circulatory system. The esoteric centre for love and compassion is often a felt experience before any of the possible somatic conditions manifest.

My heart lies bleeding
My heart is broken.

There was nothing outstanding in Mrs. K's history to indicate any gross emotional upheavals in her life but she was subject to as many daily stresses as any other human. At the time of the attack she said she 'felt that her heart was being attacked'. The heart itself was not diseased. Two things were known. Early in her life, Mrs. K. had fallen on her tail end and the curve of her coccyx was broken. She had experienced a severe heart pain thirty-five years later, which was not the result of heart disease.

The prescribed biodynamic massage was a specific move to prevent the patient from developing a somatic disorder. It was clear from Mrs. K's history that she was reasonably healthy. She felt that her life was pretty good. The wear and tear of life had been managed well. From a biodynamic point of view she had a good degree of self-regulation. During the stressful periods in her life, her harmony and balance had been adequate. Her psycho-peristalsis was active. She had, however, begun to realise that it was only as the biodynamic treatment proceeded that she realised that new feelings of well being were emerging.

Mrs. K. had no knowledge of the kundalini energy or of any other energy or movement of energy. When asked if she had felt the pain taking any particular direction she said she was not asked about this at the time of the pain episode and she did not remember. If the connection between the broken coccyx and the heart pain were a valid one then the movement of the kundalini would have been in an upward direction. In his book *Stalking the Wild Pendulum*, Itzhak Bentov[9] writes

> Only when the unfolding kundalini reaches areas of stress in the body do the symptoms become troublesome. This will then appear as localised pain. The kundalini energy continues to move on until it reaches the next stress point and the severity of the symptoms is always proportional to the degree of stress encountered.

Since the body is reflected in the cortex, we may say that the brain is also relieved of stresses. Thus the kundalini is a great stress relieving system. Once the full circuit is operating smoothly, stresses will be eliminated from the system as rapidly as they build up so that no permanent accumulation of stress is possible. Bentov notes that in some types of epilepsy, the sequence of symptoms goes in an opposite direction to the kundalini. In any epileptic attack, sensation begins in the lips, then the face, then down the neck and shoulders into the arms and legs before the motor explosion of the epileptic attack.

In the kundalini model, the energy clears the areas of over stress as it rises in the body. It then falls to return to the sacrum from whence it came. In the biodynamic model there is an upward direction to the hor-

9   Bentov, Itzhak, *Stalking the Wild Pendulum,* Destiny Books, 1977.

monic response to danger and a downward direction of the hormonic response to recovery from the stress situation. In the kundalini model, energy movement is from the sacrum and up the spine to the head. Then it descends through the head, neck, chest and abdomen and back to the sacral area.

The biodynamic theory and practice model recognises that helping the hormone responding to the physiological event can reduce over stress. The body seeks balance constantly and the appropriate biodynamic technique can help ensure the downward direction of the appropriate hormone direction. Energy Distribution massages will assist in the production of acetylcholine. Under certain circumstances there can be a clash of directional flow as appears to happen in the ileo caecal valve syndromes.[10] As long as the body is a harmoniously functioning organism, the two energetic models will work in synchrony. When the body is not functioning well, rhythms become de-synchronised. Franklyn Sills[11] describes three of these rhythms as:

> The Cranial rhythm
> The Respiratory rhythm
> The Cardiac rhythm.

The fluid factor, which was so conspicuous in Mrs K's recovery, is not covered specifically by these concepts. Mrs K. reported a prolonged flow of clear fluid from her nose. This can only be considered within the theory and concept of the chemostasis in biodynamic psychology. Dr. Randolph Stone,[12] saw the living organism in its many dimensions including the physical and the energetic. He believed in the importance of total balance in all known dimensions. In his book *The Polarity Process* Franklyn Sills gives a valuable account of the Randolph Stone principles and therapies. The life breath and organic current moves in the cerebrospinal conductor to all tissue cells and communicates with all other internal secretions and body fluids like a living cosmic breath. Dr. Stone

---

10   See Chapter 4, this Volume. The biodynamic approach to causes and treatment of idiopathic lower back pain.

11   Sills, Franklyn, *The Polarity Process,* (quoting Randolph Stone), Chapter 7, (p.127), Element Books, 1989.

12   Dr. Randolph Stone, the founder and initiator of Polarity Therapy and its principles.

saw the cerebro-spinal fluid as a vehicle for the transmission of that frequency of energy, which is light.

In *Polarity Therapy* he writes

> The cerebro-spinal fluid seems to act as a storage field and a conveyor for the ultra-sonic and the light energies.
> It bathes the spinal cord and is a reservoir for these finer energies, conducted by this fluidic medium, through all the fine nerve fibres as the first airy mind and life principles in the human body.
> Through this neuter essence, mind functions in and through matter as the light of intelligence.

On health building, Dr. Stone writes

> The CSF is the liquid medium for the life energy radiation, expansion and contraction. Where this is present there is life and healing, with normal function.
> Where this primary and essential life force is not acting in the body, there is obstruction, spasm or stagnation and pain, like gears that clash instead of meshing in their operation.

With the insights gathered from the work of Bentov,[13] Stone[14] and Sanella,[15] light was beginning to shine on Mrs. K's experience. We can say that Mrs. K's kundalini energy was moving at the time of her heart pain. It had to compromise with resistances, for example, a contracted diaphragm and a compromise would produce a less than optimum level of a feeling of well being but it was reasonably effective. Mrs. K's self-regulation was functioning well enough for her to have a reasonably healthy life. There was a reasonable balance of all functions in the body.

Along came Mrs. K's holiday. She was relaxed and comfortable. She was warm in the sun and warm and safe with her friends. This safe and secure atmosphere was exactly the kind needed to encourage a more efficient level of self-regulation. Any place in her body that needed more healthy pulsation would respond to these unaccustomed circumstances. It was as if the self-regulating rhythms in the body took an opportunistic risk and went further than ever before towards homeostasis and har-

---

13   Bentov, Itzhak, *Stalking the Wild Pendulum,* Destiny Books, 1977.
14   Sills, Franklyn, *The Polarity Process,* (quoting Randolph Stone) Element Books, 1989.
15   Sanella, Lee, *The Kundalini Experience – Psychosis or Transcendence,* Integral Publishing, California, 1987.

mony. The two areas that were less likely to have a full life pulsation, were the coccygeal fracture area and the contracted down thoracic diaphragm. When the energetic system changed at the time of the heart pain, it had been a healing crisis.

The biodynamic treatment which followed a few days after Mrs. K's return was concerned with the concept of assisting the soma to dispose of the hormonic residue which had been liberated in the crisis. The Energy Distribution massage was aimed at increasing Mrs. K's ability to relax and feel less fearful about what had happened to her. This treatment had a downward direction and intention. The venous system, together with lymph drainage would have an upward direction towards the heart in the cleansing process.

In theory this Energy Distribution Massage would conflict with upward movement of the kundalini. In the event it was possible to trust the natural sequence of energy movements which would be part of the homoeostatic move towards balance. The movement of life energy through the blood circulation pattern and the movement of the cerebro-spinal fluid through chronically depressed tissue needs a strong impetus to break through the thirty five years of the old chronic chemostasis and the resistance that this presented to energy movement.

The life energy in the kundalini and the libido energy as described by Mona Lisa Boyesen[16] originate from a common source...the cosmic source. They behave differently because they have complementary functions. Their pathways, however, are in close proximity. The biodynamic concept of the purifying functions of the plasma-faradic principle will function on all levels, for example. It may be worth mentioning that when Mrs. K. experienced the heart pain she fell to the ground.

This is one of nature's first aid methods of reducing the work that the blood circulatory system has to deal with in an emergency. There was a temporary reduction in the aortic efficiency. To remedy this, in part at least, the body needs to be horizontal. It is a biological necessity. The subsequent reduction in the blood supply to the lower limbs would make it difficult to stay upright. It has a biologic. Peace and calm and security are the important ingredients for a balanced organism.

---

16   Boyesen, Mona Lisa, 'From Libido Theory to Cosmic Energy', *Collected Papers of Biodynamic Psychology,* Chapter VII Biodynamic Psychology Publications, London, 1969-79, Reprinted from *Energy and Character*, Abbotsbury Publications.

The most obvious factor at this time of relaxation in the life of Mrs. K. was a resultant movement in all the manifestations of life energy and a very unusual amount of movement. Mrs. K.'s body would be struggling to deal with all the new movements of energy in the body. The kundalini would be reacting to the purification of tissues round the spine as a result of self-regulation. The kundalini energy would have a clearer path for its upward movement.

From a biodynamic point of view the self-regulatory mechanisms were, at least, partially liberated and the plasma-faradic function of the life energy would cleanse more tissue. This tissue which had been stagnating with chemostatic remnants (the tissue armour) would have a healthier pulsation everywhere in the body. Both of these energies having sprung from the same source are only separated by disharmonies in the organism.

The kundalini energy would continue its path upwards according to Bentov's model through the conduits of the blood vessels, particularly the aorta, and the spinal canal with all its tissues. Itzhak Bentov describes the micro-motions in the circulatory system of the blood supply from the point of view of Physics in his book *Stalking the Wild Pendulum.*[17]

The pain that Mrs.K. experienced was not difficult to understand if we consider the hypothesis of the joint action of the self-regulating function of the life energy and the plasma-faradic mechanism of purification – with the dissolution of the chemostasis in the stressed areas that were in the pathway of the kundalini energy flow. This joint action of the two aspects of life energy at this critical time would have been out of synchrony even more critically than usual as a result of the rest and relaxation Mrs. K. was taking.

The two rhythms had been in compromise for a long time. The rising kundalini which operates in more than one place at a time (theoretically, at least) would, at some point in time, find the resistance of the stasis in the diaphragm, the chemostasis. The iliac bifurcation of the aorta is at the level of the iliac crests and about the level of the third or fourth lumbar vertebra. The distance between it and the solar plexus is a matter of centimetres. There is an enormous potential for a powerful

17   Bentov, Itzhak, *Stalking the Wild Pendulum,* Destiny Books, 1977.

movement of energy between these two points if there is an unusual release of energy.

As the kundalini energy hit the solar plexus area, all the nerve tissues, autonomic as well as the central nervous system, would respond and the usual response of the central nervous system to energy meeting chemostatic abundance and resistance, is pain. Mrs. K. suffered pain in the region of the heart.

Bentov's chapter on micro motion in the body, *Sounds, Waves and Vibration*[18] provides valuable insight into what was happening in Mrs. K.'s organism. Bentov says repeatedly that the physio-kundalini is only a model and that the kundalini concept is only part of a much larger cosmic and planetary and spiritual whole. For the biodynamic therapist it has a recognisable common source with the psycho-peristalsis and its mechanisms.

Bentov's model is all about waves and resonances in the body. He describes and illustrates what happens in the largest artery of the body, the aorta, as it responds to the flow of blood from the heart. Many kinds of micro-motions are set up. These echo throughout the body from the cranial vault to the feet. Bentov describes how a standing wave occurs in the aorta, which coincides with, or is in phase with, reflected pressure pulses as a result of the movement of the aorta walls meeting the pelvic aortic bifurcation. There is, therefore, a phenomenon of the rules of physics and physiology in action.

In normal functioning, the rhythms of the heart and lungs will synchronise. It is a mechanism of the unconscious and only in the event of disturbance in the natural rhythms, will the results of the disturbance surface and the warning signs of disturbance alert the central nervous system to react...with pain. A chronic pattern of stasis needs a strong antagonist input in order to pierce through the tissue stasis. The kundalini energy and the life energy responded to the need. The two energies, nevertheless, remain phenomenological in their relationship.

From the physical viewpoint, injury to body tissue causes changes as the repair mechanisms begin. Scar tissue is not the same as the original tissue before damage occurs. Reichian principles state that an injury sustained during an emotional experience can remain in the tissues as a

---

18   Bentov, Itzhak, 'Sounds, Waves and Vibrations', Chapter 1, (p.181), *Stalking the Wild Pendulum*, Destiny Books, 1977.

memory. Work being done at the present time seems to involve memory and a connection with fluid in the synapses.[19] (See also Note at the end of this chapter.)

This would seem to have a connection with biodynamic experiences surrounding the Gerda Boyesen theory of her Deep-Draining Psycho-Postural Treatment[20] massage technique. This chemostasis occasioned by emotional or physical damage would remain in the tissue at the site of the injury until either the self-regulation mechanisms break down or, if it remains *in situ*, therapeutic intervention is needed.

In biodynamic terms we can see the broken coccyx as an impediment to a free flow of orgastic energy through the perineum. This flow which comes down the back and through the perineum and continues up the front of the body, is an important factor in providing a healthy orgastic potency, again, in biodynamic philosophy. The result of this impaired flow would contribute to psycho-pathological pressures. Mrs. K. realised that she had been marginally depressed for as long as she could remember.

Subtle Energies to be considered

In the overall view of Mrs. K's situation there is evidence of a chronic disturbance in the free flow of the life energy. There was an emotional repression, contraction and solidification in areas of her body plus the actual physical injury to the coccyx in the bone structure itself. This tissue is, by reason of its structure and its lacunae spaces, an energetic pathway. There is a factor not previously examined so far. This factor is the subtle energy field that surrounds all living tissue, and it is important in the overview of Mrs. K's condition.

This factor is complicated and complex. It is presumed to be electro-magnetic. Each cell is an electrical system. Each cell has a positive and negative property. According to Reich and Stone it has a coarse and measurable factor. The cells have an energy field. The cells in the organic systems will have composite energy fields with negative and posi-

19   Schiff, Michael, *The Memory of Water*, Thorsons, 1995.
20   See Glossary of Terms

tive poles and all these systems, whether small or large, have a potential for movement which develops into a flow.

The flow develops from areas of high excitation to areas of low excitation. As a result of this, heat or physical movement or electricity results. Stasis and paralysis of energy flow occurs when there is tissue armour or stasis and where chemostasis is the paralysing element. Mrs. K's broken coccyx would have an abnormal energy field which Stone calls a 'force field'. The chemostatic elements would result in pollution of the field. This pollution eventually pollutes the cerebro-spinal fluid and the whole of the CSF circulation as it moves through the organism.

Mrs. K. lacked a feeling of well being, although she did not know this until she had experienced therapeutic intervention after the heart pain experience. This was due to the higher centres in her mid-brain which produce the mood feeling being affected by the disturbed energy carried by the cerebro-spinal fluid. This came from the polluted energy field of the fracture in the coccyx. The cerebro-spinal fluid continues beyond the end of the spinal cord into the sacrum. The energy field of the old fracture and its chemostatic action would be reflected in the vibrational force fields, in a very subtle manner.

The cerebro-spinal-fluid is also in the minute canal of the spinal cord so the complexity of the force fields is enormous. The strong field of the chemostatically-loaded energy would be a chronically difficult pollution to absorb. This would only be possible if Mrs. K's other levels of self-regulation were in good working order and they were. When the pollution was reduced by the increased flow of life energy during the therapeutic intervention, the kundalini energy would be freed of pollution sufficiently for the mood centres to be free for fuller expression.

Mrs. K. felt her well being and realised that this was a totally new sensation. The capacity for this and the potential for further improvement were still available in spite of the chronicity of her mildly depressive state. In addition, the freeing of the thoracic diaphragm would increase the oxygenation of all the tissues including the tissues in the mid-brain where lie the mood centres. In theory, this had been a possibility.

Clinical experience subsequently showed that not all patients who had sustained fractures of the coccyx developed relevant pathologies in later life. The factor that was common to those patients who had developed pathology or idiopathic symptoms was that the damage was sustained during a highly painful emotional situation. The evidence is limited and it would not be sufficient to prove a hypothesis through these present statistics.

However, the observations are interesting and orthodoxy has not shed any light on the reason for Mrs. K's experience. Mrs. K. was the first patient warranting further study. Further encounters with patients over the years have under-lined the hypothesis that under certain circumstances a fracture of the coccyx needs more than orthopaedic attention. Some of the conditions encountered with the related life energy disturbances in different energy centres are as follows:

1. Episodic mild psychosis (Affect to the head centre)
2. Disturbances in the birthing process (Affect to sacral centre)
3. An obvious split in the appearance of the soma where the healthy-looking top half of the body was attached to a very unhealthy looking lower half from the pelvis down. Psychosexual problems were the reason for seeking therapeutic intervention. Affect to the sacral centre)
4. Migraine (Affect to the head and pelvic centre)
5. Idiopathic lower back pain with sciatic nerve involvement (Affect to sacral centre)
6. An amalgam of idiopathic disturbances – Headaches, depression, lower back pain, dysmenorrhea (Affect to the head, heart and sacral centre.)

The condition and quality of life in all patients improved after being treated with biodynamic methods and concepts. The hypothesis that the psycho-peristalsis and the kundalini energy are inter-dependent will come as no surprise to a biodynamic therapist even though the concepts are phenomenological. Medical orthodoxy has no knowledge of either concept and is in no informed or experiential position to accept either of the elements in the hypothesis.

There are other factors involved. The more that is known about the background of the patient's problem and history, the more effective will be the choices made from the basketful of biodynamic techniques. It is necessary to know as much as possible about the physical, mental, emotional and social development of the patient's condition. When this has been achieved attention has been paid and the intention of the therapeutic intervention will be that much more effective. Paying attention to the whole situation is at the very heart and foundation of all therapy. Understanding of this has to include the emerging theories of new physics.

Many of the current theories surrounding micro-vibrations, resonances and energy fields – and their effects on animal and plant organisms, verge on the phenomenal also, in fact. In practice, they are becoming part of the experiential learning of the human condition. In his book *Mind, Body and Electro-Magnetism*,[21] John Evans has pointed out

> We have moved away from the static concept of homeostasis in living organisms. Equilibrium was once thought to be controlled by the brain core. It is now recognised that there are factors that broaden the concept of this homeostasis.

Subtle measurements of the organism show that the simplistic idea of core control is too simple. The important period cycles in the body, the menstrual cycle, for instance, have more complicated rhythms than just the physiological rhythms.

Scientific attention and scrutiny currently involves observations of the electro-magnetic fields and their influences on all aspects of life. Reichian Laws are being re-assessed and given new names. Dr. Julian Kenyon[22] has a scientific study programme concerning the inter-play of the inner and outer energy fields and pathologic conditions in the human fields of psyche and soma. Harry Oldfield[23] uses a combination of physics and Kirlian concepts in psychosomatic illnesses.

In 1971 Michel Gauquelin[24] wrote his book *How Cosmic Atmosphere Energies Influence Your Health*. We live in a time of expanding insights. The role of the kundalini energy and the psycho-peristalsis phenomena in the healing process was part of my personal exploration.

The basic tenet in Biodynamic Psychology is that our exploration and subsequent treatment of any single case study begins with whatever aspect of their life needs attention. It may be that, in the first instance, they want to talk about their pain, whether it is a psychological pain, a pain in the neck, a shoulder pain, a sleeping problem or they just feel a need to talk.

21   Evans, John, *Mind, Body and Electro-Magnetism,* Element Books, 1986.
22   Kenyon, Julian, *20th Century Medicine,* British Library Catalogue, 1986.
23   Oldfield, Harry, Coghill, Roger, *The Dark Side of the Brain,* Element Books Ltd, 1988.
24   Gauquelin, Michael, *How Cosmic Atmosphere Energies Influence Your Health.* Aurora Printing, 1984.

Whatever is presented as a symptom causing most pain is that symptom to which maximum attention has to be paid. This is the most fundamental tenet in biodynamic psychology theory and practice. The pain may be physical, emotional or spiritual. The unravelling of the story of the problem begins with the first contact that the patient makes with the therapist. Mrs. K's problem manifested with a heart pain; later there was a biological unfolding of her story.

More Case Histories

1. Ann, aged 42 years, married with two teenage sons

While she was a student at a foreign university, Ann fell as she was running down some stone steps. She landed heavily on her tail end. At the time of the accident she was a long way from home and her family and she was acutely homesick. When I met Ann, it was a chance meeting and I had not expected that I would be asked to treat her. She was suffering from chronic, intractable pain in her lower lumbar and sacral region and there was severe rigidity in the area. Her medical history included having a caesarean section for the birth of each of her children. 'The birth pains just died away when I was fully dilated', she told me.

In the years following, the back pain became chronically disabling and eventually she had surgical intervention in the form of fusion of three lumbar vertebrae. The lower back pain continued. It fluctuated in intensity.

The Treatment

Ann had only one biodynamic treatment session. She lay on a mattress on the floor and I gave her an Energy Distribution massage, which seemed to be the most appropriate technique since Ann was in constant, chronic pain.

Included in the technique I introduced Passive Lifting and Opening of the Shoulder Girdle. The shoulder joints were fairly mobile, but when I attempted to open the pelvic girdle with the passive jelly-fish movements the hip joints were chronically contracted. Some patient passive jelly-fish movements in tune with her breathing pattern, resulted in some reduction in the rigid resistance in the hip joints.

I had no stethoscope with me and depended on listening for non-amplified peristaltic sounds and watching for the breath release patterns. There were some loud sounds from the gut when the muscle attachments to the bony pelvic structure were mobilised. Then Ann gave some deep breath releases.

The broken curve of the coccyx was painful at the site of the old fracture. The tissue along the coccyx curve was lumpy and the tip of the coccyx was out of reach of palpation. The psycho-peristaltic sounds were loud and explosive along the coccyx and I maintained palpation until the sounds decreased. Because I had no stethoscope I had to listen very close to Ann's abdomen. It was possible to hear loud, explosive sounds but also to identify the intermittent nature of the rather distant sounds at the beginning of treatment. After the loud explosive release sounds from the palpation of the old coccygeal fracture, the sounds became more continuous. Ann rested on her left side and said she felt sleepy. The treatment had lasted for two hours.

After the rest period, Ann was able to bend forward more comfortably and going very gently with her release breaths, she was able to bend forward so that her fingertips reached the lower third of her legs. Before treatment began, Ann had an almost totally rigid back and she would not attempt to bend forward. For impossible travel reasons this was Ann's one and only biodynamic treatment session. Three months later I heard that she had been pain free for most of this time and much more mobile. She had also experienced an increase in her vital energy.

Case history 2

H.S. is a 44-year old married woman with two daughters. She is an artist. Two years after falling heavily on the base of her spine, she began to experience periods of feeling physically ill for no discoverable medical reason. She felt ill, anxious and depressed. The acute pain in her damaged sacro-coccygeal area lasted for three months after the fall. No treatment was given at the time of the accident.

114

When I met her with a view to treating her, many things were happening in her inner life. At the time of the fall on to her spine base she was dealing with many painful problems with her children. There was a dramatic change in the way she was painting. Until recent months she had chosen gentle sea and landscapes. Suddenly she began to paint violent slashes of shapes that were dark red and dark blue almost black. The shapes slashed upwards across the paper from the left-hand corner diagonally up to the upper right-hand corner.

During the initial interview the damage to her coccyx was not mentioned. Experience has shown that this is not unusual. In the first session the frontal contractions in her body were showing clearly. Her face was tense and worried looking. Her shoulders were contracted inwards and slightly upwards. There was a slight concave bowing to the front of her body from head to pelvis. Her knees were slightly extended. The contracted shoulder girdle had produced a slight contraction in the thoracic muscles. Her breathing was shallow and a little rapid. It was necessary to reduce the concavity of the chronically flexed muscles at the front of her body. An Energy Distribution massage was indicated.

During the first part of the treatment H. lay on her back. The peristaltic sounds were rather distant and only intermittent. Some passive lifting of the whole of her right arm produced a few explosive sounds but these subsided. By this time I was alert to the possibility of damage to the lower spine and I asked H. if she had at any time had a fall. She then remembered falling and landing on her lower spine, two years previously. At the time the pain was severe but over the months, it diminished and receded. At the end of the treatment session, H. said she felt strong streamings down her arms and legs.

Therapy continued in a somewhat piecemeal fashion. H. had three treatments from me and then was treated by a therapist who lived much nearer. This therapist was shown how the therapy was designed and why. Over the following months the therapist continued the pattern of treatments and the results of the therapy were very positive. When possible I was also able to give H. some treatments.

Several times the treatments had touched areas of sadness and had released deep crying. These released feelings were always followed by H. feeling streamings down her legs and feelings of lightness. The depressive feelings, feelings of extreme weariness and feeling ill all receded. Her work expanded joyfully as did her artistic expression. The violent colours have given way to big, blooming, colourful and uninhibited flower studies in pinks and reds.

Currently, H. paints impressionistic pictures of dancers and dancing movements. Her landscapes are also of uninhibited, colourful but blended soft colours. The pain in the coccyx area has almost gone. The fact that treatment began only two years after the injury was sustained was an obvious factor in her good recovery. It is still necessary from time to time to empty the coccygeal area in order to free the tissue of any accumulated chemostasis. It was very interesting to see the therapy in terms of the colours changing from the murky black and red to crimson and pinks.

Case History 3

T. aged thirty two. An unmarried woman, no children, with a history of two surgical terminations of pregnancies. T. had fallen from a horse in her early adolescence and landed on her sacrum. Her subsequent development during her adolescence was marked by her angry relationship with her parents, particularly with her father and this had been an ongoing situation even before the accident. Her father had died when she was in her late twenties and she continued to have strong feelings of resentment against him after death. She and her mother continued a very volatile relationship.

T. sought help through psychotherapy and bioenergetics after the death of her father. She was a bright intelligent woman and much of her wit was spent in manipulating all relationships including most of the therapists she consulted. The manipulation was generally sexual. Her appearance was at first glance more male the female. She had a shortish stocky body, very short hair, not much breast development, a swaggering walk and she generally wore mannish trousers and shirts.

Once or twice a year she suffered from transient, mild near psychotic episodes. They were mild in that they never lasted for more than a few days and then just went away. An attack felt to her like a sudden deep and black depression. There was a fear with horror. The attacks came in the night and she would be so frightened that she would ring

116

round the family for someone to be with her in the very acute times of the attack. There was panic and fear and horror, then it would subside and disappear. There was no apparent triggering factor.

She came for a relaxation treatment. She said she felt tensions in her body that were uncomfortable and were becoming more and more a barrier to relaxation. Early in the therapeutic process I found historical and physical evidence of a broken coccyx. There was evidence that this had been sustained at a time when her father had been very angry with her for hanging round street corners and staying out very late. She was about fifteen years old and had had several sexual encounters.

She experienced some relaxation in the Energy Distribution massage. Although there were obvious breath releases there was very little psycho-peristaltic activity. Periosteal massage to the sacro-coccygeal junction produced deep crying followed by loud explosive psychoperistaltic sounds and deeper breath release patterns. The fracture was about two centimetres along the coccygeal curve. This was very painful when pressure was applied but as the peristaltic sounds increased, the pain lessened. The tip of the coccyx was out of reach of palpation. The thoracic diaphragm was still very contracted.

As she lay prone, I applied some pulsatory touch to the upper thoracic area with both hands. After some thirty seconds she gave some very deep breath releases. As the lower thoracic area expanded it was possible to see that there was very little reciprocal movement in the pelvic area and this reflected the tensions there. At the end of the session she said she was feeling profoundly weary.

A week later there was very little feedback. Energy Distribution was used together with a very gentle, passive, jelly-fish technique to reduce the tensions in the pelvic musculature. There was resistance to the opening of the pelvic girdle in the right leg when it was at an angle of forty-five degrees. I stayed with the resistance. There was some trembling in the limb and then the leg relaxed. The angle widened and T. gave a big release breath accompanied by increased peristaltic sounds. These sounds were short lived.

T. was having analytic psychotherapy twice weekly elsewhere. I made a contract with her that I would work with the biodynamic body techniques and not the psychotherapy. This did not mean that I would ignore any psychological reactions to what we were doing together or any abreactive responses. If they occurred total attention would be paid to these responses. I was primarily interested in the impact on the whole of the organism. Boundaries, however, were a necessary part of the therapeutic process. Experience had shown that dangers in the transference process could be enhanced when the patient is having two or more different therapeutic disciplines at the same time. Clear boundaries are helpful to both patient and therapist.

T.'s chaotic psychological development caused most of her painful problems. It seemed that the pain and grief and anger needed many kinds of expressions. There was anger throughout her organism. There was suppressed grief and guilt in the terminations of her pregnancies and there was deep emotional and spiritual pain echoing throughout her physical body.

She began to add together her understanding of her physical pain with the deeper dimensions of the emotional and spiritual pain. I used the Energy Distribution and Emptying techniques. She had five more treatment sessions and during that time there was no more deep crying or any vegetative releases of any magnitude. On two occasions she needed to go to the bathroom to pass urine. She remarked that it was hot. Her breathing was fuller and deeper. The whole of her chest moved in her breathing and there was an increase in the pelvic movements in response.

Throughout the six weeks of therapy I used the gentle touch technique, the Pulsatory Touch, incorporating it into the general Energy Distribution technique. It was very effective and productive of good peristaltic sounds indicating release of tissue tensions. T. always, in the latter treatments, responded with release breaths and always reported feeling more relaxed. This gentle touch technique was applied as T. lay prone with her head turned towards her right. I sat at the head of the massage table and as T. breathed in, I met the in-breath with my hands on each side of the upper thoracic back muscles.

I continued the pulsatory touch, lifting my hands with the in-breath and applying gentle pressure down with the out-breath; continuing this rhythmic touch for several minutes. As soon as the peristaltic sounds became more continuous or the release breaths came more easily, I then applied long effleurage strokes to the whole length of the back in a downward direction which is the direction of the Energy Distribution technique.

T. decided that she would stop the body therapy and continue to have her Jungian therapy. She had received six biodynamic treatments at weekly intervals. At the end of this time there was a freer flow of energy through the sacrum and coccyx. Stasis was reduced. The old fracture site was painful at the beginning of the course of treatment and pain free at the end of the six weeks. T. was aware that she could return to me at any time the need was there.

I saw her again a year later. In the meantime she had had no further massage therapy. I was surprised to see so many changes in her. Her stocky figure had slimmed down and she had grown her hair to a shoulder length style. She looked very feminine and wore soft flowing clothes. Her voice was less strident and I gathered that she had a gentle relationship with a new man. Her terror attacks had not returned.

Case History 4

J. A single woman, thirty years old. No children and no history of her ever having been pregnant. She was seeking help in dealing with the effects of an over-stressed life style. She was a high-powered executive in the rag trade. She said she suffered from tense, nervous headaches.

She was also concerned and anxious about her inability to maintain a strong loving relationship. She thought she loved her present partner but was unable to understand why she needed to fight with him so much. Her history revealed a difficult relationship with her mother. J. was one of the very few people seeking help, who recalled the time when she fell and broke her coccyx. This she recalled at the time of her interview: At the age of twelve, after a quarrel with her mother she defiantly slid down the wooden banisters outside her apartment home.

Her mother shouted at her that it was dangerous and that she should stop being silly. The staircase was an open one in a large expensive block of flats. They lived on the first floor. While still angry with her mother she did fall and landed on the bottom marble step. She recalled the acute pain in her lower spine and the feeling of fear. She was frightened by the fall and also the fear of what her mother would say. She thought that she did not tell her mother that she had fallen, or even that her mother was there when she fell. She had no treatment for the pain, which she thought lasted some weeks.

Her body patterns were remarkable. Her top half was well proportioned and beautiful but below the pelvis her thighs and lower legs were thick and though well shaped, they looked lifeless and hypotonic. The skin was very dry. The tissue was inelastic and finger pressure left shallow dents, indicating stagnation of tissue fluid – chemostasis. The colour of her lower limbs was grey and contrasted with the pink tones of her upper body. She said she could never walk far without her legs feeling weary.

Therapy was directed at changing the energy flow and so balancing the two halves of her body. She was full of resentments. She had a prestigious career in fashion and loved it, but she felt dissatisfied with her life. J. talked for most of the first session and I explained to her how I saw what was happening in her body and the possible influence of the damaged coccyx. The Energy Distribution technique was used from the beginning, but I did not touch the area of fracture for two weeks. I wanted to change the fluid situation, or at least influence it, particularly in her lower limbs.

I started by using a fast up-going petrissage treatment for a few minutes on each leg. There was no psycho-peristalsis. This was followed by an Energy Distribution massage. After six weeks of combined massage and psychotherapy, there were notable changes. The hypotonic tissue became more elastic and the pitting was less on applying finger pressure. The colour of the tissue was less grey.

J. said she felt less tired and was feeling lighter. The tissues of her upper thighs produced quite large lumpy residual nodules in the deep dermal tissues. These responded to a firm emptying touch with loud mixed sounds. J. took a stethoscope home with her so that she could continue the emptying of the tissue between treatments and also to get some positive feedback while she listened to her gut sounds, which she found enthralling. Her boyfriend also came for some relaxation treatment and to express how he felt. At this point, two months into the therapeutic process, she was offered an exciting job in the United States and it would be possible for them to go together. She said: 'At last I've made a decision without dithering'.

The therapy had been mixed and truly biodynamic. The Energy Distribution technique was very valuable in the first treatments. J. was very angry with life and she needed time and some evidence of change before she could trust. She was able to contribute to these changes by continuing the emptying of the upper thigh tissues. The chemostatic problems were most noticeable below the pelvic area, so it was good to mobilise the tissue so that the blood circulation pattern helped to carry the life energy through the areas of stasis. There was considerable stasis in the gluteals and some vital mobilisation was imperative before treatment at the site of the old fracture was begun. The emptying of the tissue stasis in the coccyx was achieved by deep periosteal touch together with work with the biofield.

The stethoscope is the monitoring tool and when the sounds took longer to emerge it paid to wait and not move on too quickly. Psychotherapy was, in general, directed at encouraging J. to express her resentments and when these were spilling over into the body she kicked her way through her rage while lying on the mattress. In the short time that we worked together, she needed plenty of encouragement so that after each session she found a place in her body that felt good.

Her independent well being was beginning to emerge and she felt she knew and understood more about herself than before the therapy began. J.'s insight into being able to make a decision is a common experience amongst people who have damage to the pelvic area. Decisions may be made in the head, but if the pelvis does not move there is a problem. The pelvic area is the place that allows forward movement and stasis in this area will contribute to the difficulties of making and carrying out decisions. The pelvic area is the going centre.

Case History 5

L. A woman of thirty-eight years, happily married with two small sons eight and six years old. There had been birthing problems and a very prolonged labour in both confinements. Each confinement ended with a forceps delivery. She was, now, seeking help for an acute neck and shoulder pain. Physiotherapy had only been of temporary help. She was afraid that nothing could help her and she resisted taking even mild painkillers. L. said she suffered from migrainous headaches. She also had considerable discomfort from a chronic lower back pain with some sciatic nerve involvement in the right leg down to the calf muscles. L's neck and shoulder pain were the most uncomfortable symptoms, though she found sitting in the evening was difficult because the sciatic nerve pain was distressing.

L. had damaged her coccyx and lower spine when she fell from a swing at the age of twelve. Her family life at that time was unhappy as a result of her quarrelling parents. She does not recall much happiness in her childhood. The therapeutic process began with an Energy Distribution massage. She said the whole of her body felt tense. In fact, much of her musculature was hypotonic. There were muscle tensions and contractions in her scalp, and in her neck and head. Her eyes were clouded with not much life in them although she was cheerful and she smiled a lot. Her lower back was rigid and contracted in the lumbo-sacral area.

The treatment would be directed at reducing the tensions in her body as much as possible and to palpate the coccygeal area at an early stage. It was grossly distorted as a result of the old injury. It was very long and the fracture had caused the coccyx to have a right-angled bend. The tip of the coccyx was inaccessible, lying deep in the gluteal fold. It was excruciatingly tender and I had to stop even the most careful touch to the periosteum because the pain made L. contract in a startle.

After the initial treatment had been completed L. turned over on to her left side. She said she was feeling relaxed and felt sleepy in spite of the sharpness of the coccygeal pain. The psycho-peristaltic sounds were flowing freely and were a mixture of explosive and watery sounds. As she lay over on her left side I used the bio-field in the area of the gluteal cleft to contact the coccyx in the fracture area. The sounds changed as my hand was about ten centimetres away from the body. I began to pull at the bio-field with her in-breaths. Her diaphragm released a big breath and the sounds were loud and explosive. I worked in this way for about fifteen minutes and used this technique whenever I treated her.

Attention and pressure to the inter-phalangeal neck reflex of the right big toe proved to be a significant item in the therapeutic repertoire. Thereafter she could use this massage of her big toe to help her neck pain by using this reflex correspondence for herself and feel able to take some responsibility for reducing her discomforts. She continued to receive Energy Distribution massage together with regular emptying of the fracture area. The acute pain did not recur with that initial violence.

Mobilisation of the muscle groups involved in her breathing patterns were attended to each time, together with mobilisation of the pelvic musculature and stretching of the lumbar musculature. At the end of four months of weekly treatments the sciatic nerve pain and the migrainous headaches had gone. Pain in the coccyx area varied. Sometimes it was totally pain free and then for no apparent reason it would be painful and the rigidity and contraction in the lower lumbar area would appear.

A year later her neck and shoulder pain is far less frequent and disabling and she does not feel trapped inside an unending pain. She has learned to relax her neck and shoulders and to control the pain in her lower back with gentle stretching exercises. Her eyes are constantly bright. She is a businesswoman and cares for a growing family very successfully. Exacerbation of the pains in her body recur when she is overtired and in need of a holiday. These pains are always easier to remove when her coccyx is free from pain. An interesting aspect is that before she had treatment and while she was still in pain somewhere in her body, she was taking driving lessons and was looking forward to having her own car.

Although, in theory, she was ready to take her road test, she told me: 'I never felt that I was in control through my behind'. This was irrelevant at first glance. After four months of treatment she decided to take her test. She passed and thoroughly enjoys her freedom through being able to drive. L. is aware that she may need maintenance treatment from time to time and can anticipate when extra stress will produce the pain for which she may need help. At no time has she produced symptoms of great sadness or anger and the hypotonicity of her muscles seems to be her barometer of her emotional life.

Summary

Conclusions are hard to come by and it has been a long haul since I met Mrs. K. and her heart pain. I have to thank her for the valuable additions to my biodynamic experience, as we all constantly search for understanding of what it is like to be human. No new techniques were needed.

Biodynamic principles and techniques provided a comprehensive basket from which appropriate tools could be chosen. From a scientific point of view the number of cases were far too small to merit conclusions.

However, there were consistencies in the observations and responses to treatment and these consistencies continue to be present in other patients who have developed psychosomatic conditions following damage to the coccygeal area of the spine. The most consistent observation is that the patient who has sustained an injury to the coccyx while under severe emotional upheaval is more likely to develop psychosomatic or idiopathic conditions. I believe that more investigation will provide more valuable understanding of other conditions such as Parkinson's Disease or Multiple Sclerosis.

Note: Reference: *The Memory of Water*, Michael Schiff.

> Clinically, water seems to have a memory for past exposures to highly coherent frequencies that have taken place since it was last distilled. Apart from the clinical effects described above, some degree of laboratory demonstration is possible.

This main article[25] seems to explain current theories about fluid in biodynamic terms. It is helpful to look at current work. For instance, Michel Schiff in his book *The Memory of Water*[26] reviews the Benvenista controversy on the memory of water after homeopathic memories were completely eradicated. Michel Schiff's book clarifies the argument somewhat. Jacques Benvenista is the respected French scientist who directed a research team for over four years in order to study the ability of water to remember previous contacts. The team achieved several breakthroughs in this study.

An article was published in *Nature* with the findings of the research team. Reactions to publication were very violent. The relevance to the neuro-physiology of the synapse is that it is difficult for neuro-scientists to do any lateral thinking. Nevertheless the current controversies about water memory can be linked to what we have experienced in the biody-

25 Smith, Cyril, and Best, Simon, *Electromagnetic Man*, Chapter 6, (p. 99), J.M. Dent and Sons Ltd., Bath Press, Avon, 1990
26 Benveniste, Jacques, in *Nature*, 1988.

namic deep-draining psycho-postural treatment massage, whereby, for example, old viral conditions have reappeared after this treatment, as part of a cleansing process, prior to being eliminated from the body naturally.

It is possible that the chemostatic fluid, the tissue fluid, in the environment of countless synapses in the human organism can be explained by applying Reichian laws to the equation and therefore this is very bio-dynamic in practice.

The Nervous System

Neuro-physiology describes the synapse as a gap between one nerve cell (neurone) terminal and another, adjacent, contiguous neurone. It is an electrical system and a biochemical system and only nerve cells have synapses. The moving nerve impulses through the axon, i.e. sodium ions, have a positive electrical charge. It is possible that the Reichian Law will apply here but we need more knowledge.

Probably (!) the positive ion will attract water (the thunder storm) and if there is an area in the body, the diaphragm for instance, where the ionic balance mechanism will be disturbed, then more of the chemostatic quality of the water will change the balance. The inter-flow of electrical charge would be affected and the electrical situation would affect not only the neurones but also the tissue involved.

CHAPTER 6

Biodynamic concepts and treatment in the idiopathic pathology of Parkinson's Syndrome

This chapter attempts to orientate the biodynamic treatment of the Parkinson's[1] disorder and to describe the relevant touch techniques in the psychosomatic manifestation of the patient's condition. Parkinsonism is the name given to a clinical syndrome that includes the apparent impairment of voluntary movements of the body's peripheral musculature. Rigidity and tremor are the most obvious symptoms. The condition occurs in approximately 1 in 1000 of the population. The incidence rises to 1 in 100 in those people over 60 years of age.

Many patients who suffer from Parkinson's disorder may also show evidence of cerebral atherosclerosis. It is not clear whether these two conditions occur co-incidentally. Tremor is the condition for which the patient initially seeks advice. At first it affects the fingers and then the muscles of the forearm. It happens when the fingers are at rest though purposive movement tends to reduce the shaking.

Rigidity may be experienced early in the development of the syndrome and resistance to the passive movement of the joints and flexion of the neck, hips, elbows and knees can be observed. The gait is characteristic, with short steps and a developing shuffle mode of walking. The facial muscles become slow in re-acting to emotional expression and develop a mask-like appearance. Speech may change in character as the muscles necessary for speech are involved in the syndrome.

---

[1]   James Parkinson, a London physician, published his findings in the treatment of the neurological disorder in six patients during the second decade of the nineteenth century. A hundred years later an American physician named Rowntree linked the name of Parkinson with the condition known as *Paralysis Agitans*.

The hypothesis leading to biodynamic treatment of the Parkinson's Syndrome

Each patient referred for biodynamic treatment suffered from excessive rigidity of the neck and shoulder muscles and together with this somatic symptom there was in every referred case a history of deep, severe but unexpressed grief. This rigidity was the result of the enormous muscular power needed to control the expression of grief and affected the diaphragm, the thoracic muscles and the cervical musculature. The strong and chronic contractions of the muscles would result in an inefficient blood flow to the contents of the skull. Poor oxygenation of these tissues would be inevitable

My hypothesis was that an increased, healthy blood supply to the whole of the body, but most particularly to those areas reflecting cerebral inefficiency, could be achieved by using the concepts and techniques of biodynamic psychology. A freer blood supply to the mid-brain could perhaps influence the idiopathic degeneration associated with the Parkinson's syndrome. I have seen and treated far too few patients suffering from Parkinson's syndrome to make a scientific analysis, but certainly enough to see improvements in the quality of life for every one treated.

The Case History of Ann

Ann, aged 67 years, had been diagnosed as suffering from Parkinson's Disease. She had begun experiencing the first signs of her condition a year and a half after the death of her much loved son. She is a secretive woman, unused to revealing her inner feelings. Expressions of grief were private and in secret, and this was also reflected within the marriage. She told me: 'We didn't come together to share the grief of losing him. He (her husband) hates anything emotional'.

After the neurologist had made the diagnosis, Ann told her husband but she did not tell anybody else. Her response to the diagnosis was a painful mixture of fear, that she would end up in a wheelchair, inevitably, and shame that she had a shameful disease that would deprive her of any control over her body or mind. She felt hopeless and helpless and an increasingly depressive state was a further burden.

It became more and more difficult to rouse herself to begin the day, and she saw little point in any of the daily routines that made up her life. Grief, fear and painful depression were the over-riding feelings and these contributed to an increasing immobility. Ann was in physical and psychological pain. A caring and observant friend confronted Ann and persuaded her to share what was happening.

This led to my first meeting with her and the beginning of an exploratory journey together. The initial therapeutic relationship was very difficult for Ann. 'I was talked into this', she said and her tone was both resigned and resentful. She expressed doubt that there was anything that would help her; her fate was sealed. Her husband drove her from their home as Ann does not drive. She got out of the car unaided and her husband, addressing his wife, said: 'I will pick you up in an hour and a half' and then disappeared. It was clear that Ann did not find getting out of the car too difficult, but as she took her first steps it was obvious that her gait was not natural. She had a limp and her posture was too upright.

The Consultation

Ann was reluctant to talk about anything that may have shed some light on her medical history. As a result of her difficulties I confined the quest for information to the simplest and least provocative questions. I had seen that she had a limp and I asked her where in her body she felt pain. This was for her an acceptable line of enquiry and she began to talk about the pains in her body. There were places that were constantly painful such as her left shoulder and her right hip. The pain seemed to be worse when she got up in the morning. Some four years previously Ann had fallen downstairs and from her description of her injuries she had partially dislocated her shoulder joint. No bones had been broken but probable damage to the joint capsule was the consequence.

As a result of increasing osteoarthritis in her right hip Ann had had a hip replacement two years later. She said that there had been severely painful osteoarthritis for a long time before the operation. Ann found it easy to talk about the many physical pains she suffered daily, but apart from this she shied away from anything to do with her Parkinson's symptoms. The consultation was prolonged and I was able to observe and pay attention to the way Ann was.

The overall impression was of a sad, depressed and overweight woman who was not meeting her future with anything positive. We discussed Ann's medication but she was unclear about the dosage of each drug. She thought that she was taking something for her depression and for the symptoms of Parkinsonism.

I outlined the therapeutic programme we could follow together. This would be to address whatever was uppermost in her discomfort at each session and we agreed to an initial contract of four sessions of therapy on a weekly basis. Ann was a little hesitant to respond positively but this turned out to be because she had to be sure that the plan did not interfere with her husband's golf fixtures.

Treatments

It was uncomfortable for Ann to undress and get on to the massage table but I was anxious to see, even with help, what her physical difficulties were and there were many. Ann found it impossible to lie on her back without the support of at least three pillows to raise her head and shoulders. This was almost entirely due to the very contracted neck musculature and because she felt dizzy without the pillow support.

This treatment session was all about getting to know each other. I wanted to know a great deal about Ann and her pain. Ann had retained most of her clothing and I found initial difficulty finding a responsive place for my electronic stethoscope. Energy Distribution massage was indicated in order that Ann might feel something happening. Assessing the tensions in her body and paying attention to them with touch could dissipate at least some of the superficial contractions. There were good psycho-peristaltic sounds almost at once. The sounds were of good volume and continuous.

I began the massage by working on Ann's face and head. Time was running out and Ann was anxious not to keep her husband waiting. On the other hand I was intent on completing enough of the treatment session to get an overall picture of Ann's needs and not in participating in the hurry and hustle, which would result in more startle patterns developing. Ann's hair was thin and the scalp muscles were tense and rigid. As the tissues were mobilised, the sounds from the scalp were loud and explosive. Over the forehead the skin was dry and flaky. Ann's makeup was important to her and she wore mascara and a very bright lipstick which I tried to avoid touching. The whole of her facial structure was touched and responded with loud mixed sounds from the stethoscope.

Gentle lifting was applied to her right shoulder. It was not painful but it was rigid. There was an obvious tremor in her right hand and the fingers were thickened and stiff with some clawing. The right wrist and all the fingers were gently mobilised and stretched. The elbow was mobilised in the same way. Firm petrissage to the whole of the tissues of the right arm in an upward direction produced loud sounds from the stethoscope. Long effleurage strokes from the shoulder joint to the fingertips completed the treatment of the right arm.

The left shoulder was stiff and painful and the elbow joint was slightly bent in contraction though there was no history of damage to this joint. There was a noticeable area of dry scaliness over the mid-humerus. The left shoulder joint was lifted and mobilised in tune with the breath pattern; lifting with the in-breath and allowing the arm to drop gently on the out-breath. The upper arm tissues were also mobilised, the musculature being lifted away from the bony shaft of the humerus.

There was a strong psycho-peristaltic response from the area of dryness over the mid-humerus and a patch of hyperaemia[2] appeared over the site. This response to this area has been noted in those patients being treated in a biodynamic way for Parkinson's syndrome. The area of dryness of the skin seems to follow the anterior branch of the *profunda brachii* artery and the peripheral radial nerve and perhaps, an acupuncture point. It could be that the energy is withdrawn to bone level at this point. Validation for this hypothesis could only come if it were known why the area is so affected and if awareness and treatment influence positive improvement in the patient's neuropathy. Perhaps the acupuncture point is the clue. The continuation of the artery into the humeral circumflex vessel and then into the arterial blood supply to the brain is, possibly, noteworthy.

The treatment to Ann's left arm followed the pattern of touch that had been used on her right arm. The fingers of the left hand were thick-

2   See Glossary of Terms.

ened with osteoarthritic changes in the joints and some clawing. The tissues of the whole arm from the fingers upward to the shoulder joint were firmly mobilised in an upward direction. There is a certain minimal encouragement for the lymph system to be influenced by mobilising the tissue in this way. Energy Distribution strokes from the shoulder joint to the toes completed the treatment to the left arm. These strokes from the shoulders to the toes are important because they give a feeling to the patient that all of the body is having attention.

Ann's breathing was shallow and there was no pelvic movement in response to the breaths; neither was there any movement in the mid and lower abdomen. I had, at first, tried to place the head of the stethoscope under her lower lumbar region, there was so much muscular contraction in the lower back, however, that it was necessary to find another area so the stethoscope head was placed over the upper abdomen.

The skin over Ann's thighs and upper third of the lower legs was smooth and warm. The lower leg areas and the ankles showed increasing dryness and immobility of the skin. The feet were excessively dry and both soles were thickened and cracked. A common impression in those patients suffering from Parkinsonism is that there is a withdrawal of energy from the periphery. This leads to a therapeutic need, not only to distribute the stuck energy, wherever it may be, but to make sure that the periphery of the body should have particular attention paid to the head, hands and feet.

Why does this happen? Why does the energy appear to go into the body depths? Ann complained that she was always very depressed in the mornings whether she had slept or not. She was also compelled to rise slowly because she felt very dizzy. Ann felt cumbersome and this made the next task of turning over on the massage table formidable. Achievement of the prone position was a major accomplishment. The stiffness of her neck was a problem and she could only tolerate this position by lying at an incline with three pillows to support her upper body and with her arms supporting her head. The stiffness of the whole of her body was marked and the massage treatment consisted of mobilising the muscles of her back, her buttocks and her legs.

Ann refused to rest after the treatment. On being helped off the table she felt very dizzy and it was necessary to wait until this feeling lessened. In spite of the difficulties of getting on and off the table and the lengthy interview and treatment session, Ann said she felt different, not better but different.

More about Parkinsonism

In current medical terms Parkinsonism is, perhaps, better defined as a collection of clinical features that are seen by the diagnosticians as having a commonality. The condition is caused by a degeneration of the basal ganglia. The basal ganglia is the name given to the areas of grey matter at the base of the cerebral cortex.

This area consists of the *globus pallidus*, the *corpus striatum*, the *substantia nigra* and the *sub-thalamic nucleus*. The disease is associated with an increase in muscle tone in both extensor and flexor muscles so that the patient has difficulty in moving about by means of any voluntary muscle activity. The main pathological feature of Parkinsonism is the loss of the neuro transmitter Dopamine. Parkinsonism, as a result of arterio-sclerotic changes is reported to appear at a later stage in a patient's life.

Some alternative causes of Parkinsonism

> Drugs, e.g., of the Phenothiazine group
> Head injury (e.g., boxing)
> Carbon Monoxide poisoning
> Tumours
> Hysteria
> Alcohol poisoning
> Extra-pyramidal disturbance in patients with diffuse vascular disease
> Slow virus infection.

In the development of the disorder there may be an insidious manifestation with a gap in the presentation of symptoms of two or three years. In the case of drug induced or post-encephalitic cases the presentation of the symptoms may be more rapid. In most cases of Parkinsonism the tremor is the first symptom. It begins in the first fingers then moves into the arms.

Later on, the tremor affects the tongue and legs. The tremor is slow and in the earliest stages involves rhythmical movement of the thumb towards the fingers. The tremor occurs with the limb at rest and lessens with purposive movement. Stress and embarrassment aggravate the tremor's amplitude. Head tremors occur rarely, although in one patient there was a concomitant tick involving the muscles of the face and neck and jaw muscles and a deep psychological dilemma and pain. As rigidity of the musculature increases the tremor may diminish.

The cog wheel phenomenon, a super-imposed jerky sensation, may occur. Fine movements may become increasingly difficult and there may be a noticeable loss of arm swinging. The normal gait progresses into short, shuffling steps. Slow walking is often accompanied by periods of uncontrolled acceleration while going downhill. This is called festination. Falls are common. Speech can be affected with loss of voice volume.

Emotional facial response can be slow and there may be impaired pupillary accommodation. Strong fear or anger may, temporarily, overcome the hyperkinesis (the impairment of voluntary movement). There may be changes in the size and quality of the patient's handwriting. Fine movements necessary for feeding and the fastening of clothing buttons is impeded and very slow. A dorsal kyphosis, causing a stooped posture, may also occur.

Medical Treatment

The medical treatment of the condition aims at replacing the missing dopamine through biochemical agents. Most commonly L.dopa in combination with dopa-decarboxylase inhibitor and anti-cholinergic agents and a direct dopaminergic agent such as bromocryptine is prescribed. The condition warrants physiotherapy, which is palliative.

Direct intervention to the affected mid-brain area is being researched and attempted. Introducing heat, alcohol and, currently, relevant embryonic tissue into the crucial area has been tried with very mixed results.

Lars Olson and colleagues of the Karolinska Institute in Stockholm did the first neural transplants on human beings. They transferred chromaffin cells from the adrenal medulla to the brain in a number of patients with severe Parkinson's disease. Of the two patients treated with the experimental surgery, one showed significant improvement and no deterioration in the condition of the other patient. In the analysis of the minute cell function of the chromaffin cell it is reported that:

> One step in the synthesis of adrenalin, the transformation of dopamine into nor adrenalin, takes place inside the vesicle. It is catalysed by a four-part enzyme, dopamine betahydroxylase, with ascorbic acid as a co-factor.

In the process, the ascorbic acid loses an electron and becomes semi-hydroascorbate. A third protein in the vesicle membrane, cytochrome B561, transfers electrons (e-) into the vesicles from a complementary process in the cystol, thereby renewing the ascorbic acid and enabling the synthesis of nor adrenalin to proceed.

This work on the importance of the chromaffin cell was reported by Stephen W. Carmichael and Hans Winkler.[3] They describe how the flight or fight response to danger floods the blood with adrenalin at three hundred times the normal concentration. This is the result of an excretory event in the adrenal medulla. Chromaffin cells manufacture, store and secrete a complexity of hormones the most important of which is adrenalin.

The importance of this research is obvious. It is not only important that the bio-chemical minutiae have been revealed, but it is at the minutiae end of the therapeutic intervention that changes must take place if there is to be a reversal or halt in the progress to more pathology.

The Biodynamic perspective of Parkinson's disease

An idiopathic disorder is described as such because there is no apparent predisposing cause for the condition. When biodynamic concepts and treatment are introduced in to the way the pathological situation has developed, it may be possible to view the total organism in another way and, perhaps in a fresh light. There is no biodynamic conceptual approach to this disorder in a scientific study as far as I can establish.

---

3   Research by Carmichael Stephen W., and Winkler, Hans, 'Chromaffin Cells', *Scientific American*, August 1985.

This chapter is, therefore, based on anecdotal case histories. The use of the stethoscope is important to monitor the sounds coming from the gut as the therapeutic techniques are used. The Gerda Boyesen concept of the role of the gut in the digestion of the residual stress products is the basis for much of the treatment of psychosomatic conditions. It is also valid to point out the value of bioenergetic concepts as conceived by Wilhelm Reich.

One of Reich's concepts was that of Cosmic Law 1.[4] This states that where there was a strong energy field it would attract water. These concepts of Gerda Boyesen[5] and Wilhelm Reich are officially still in the realm of phenomenology, but in biodynamic treatments we have been using them usefully for over three decades.

We listen to the amazing variety of sounds from the gut and we see changes in the patient we are treating. The patient begins to be aware of changes in the way they feel physically and psychologically. The biodynamic therapist should be aware of the treatment prescribed by the patient's medical practitioners.

Dialogue between the therapist and the patient's family doctor is necessary if symptoms arise in the course of treatments which, if the therapist considers them relevant to medically prescribed drugs – for instance, should be communicated to the doctor. The patients I have treated and referred to in this article have been elderly and severely depressed. Who would not be depressed if given the diagnosis of Parkinsonism?

The patient is often prescribed an anti-depressant along with the drugs to treat the symptoms of the disorder. The depressive state can be painfully destructive of the feeling of well being. Many patients could not remember when they last felt pleasurable excitement. All the patients I treated had been depressed for a long time before the first symptoms appeared.

4   Wilhelm Reich, Cosmic Law I and II [ORI and II] from *Energy & Character* Volume 6, No. 2, 1975. Cosmic Law 1 stipulates that where there is a strong energy field it will attract a weaker energy field. Cosmic Law 2 states that fluid attracts energy, and energy attracts fluid.

5   Boyesen, Gerda, and Boyesen, Mona Lisa, 'Psycho-Peristalsis', Part IV, *Collected Papers of Biodynamic Psychology*, Volumes 1 and 2, Biodynamic Psychology Publications, London, 1969-79.

Three of the patients had suffered the tragic loss of a beloved child under shocking circumstances. Another patient nursed his wife through her illness and eventual death from cancer. She and he had struggled through great difficulties to reach a plateau of calm and peace in their marriage. Then she died. He found it difficult to express either grief or his rage.

A further patient, now in his late sixties, had worked hard all his life to rise above the spiritual and physical poverty of his childhood. He reached a high level of success in a very competitive industry. He retired and looked forward to sharing time and aesthetic pleasures and travel with his wife. She died at this time. The grief of these people was followed within two years by the first symptoms of Parkinsonism.

Grief as a catalyst

It would seem from the past history of each of these people that either they were not able to express their grief at the time or that the grief was only partially expressed. This would result in a retained emotional, and therefore hormonal, reaction in the thoracic diaphragm. In biodynamic terms the startle pattern occasioned by the loss and grief was incomplete. The out-breath completion had been inhibited. The diaphragm acts as a controller of emotion and literally cuts the flow of energy in half.

The Gerda Boyesen concept of life energy transported through the blood supply is clearly evident in Ann's body. The shock of the loss can seem to be a threat to the very life of the person who grieves. The essential self of the grieving person is threatened. The shock of the loss inhibits the breath. The pain is held in check by the contraction of the diaphragm. If it is not held it may annihilate the self.

This is the biological importance of the flight or fight mechanism of the hormonal startle pattern. According to biodynamic principles and confirmed constantly by our clinical findings, an emotional stasis in the thoracic diaphragm will affect the pelvic movements.

As Dr. Eva Reich[6] has taught, this pelvic hammock containing the very important pelvic organs behaves, in health, in synchrony with the thoracic diaphragm. Deep within the lower pelvis lies the individual's

6   Eva Reich, MD. – daughter of Wilhelm Reich.

centre of gravity. This is the place of the essential self. This is the place of the esoteric hara.

One aspect of the grief phenomena is whether it involves retainment or containment. Superficially, the two terms mean more or less the same. In biodynamic terms they can have important though subtle difference. Retained grief has to some extent denied the need to grieve, so the person's release of rage and fear is incomplete. The natural move towards balance and homeostasis is damaged. The psycho-peristalsis is inhibited and chronic retention of the hormonic startle remnants is the result.

The biodynamic therapies help the vegetative nervous system to complete the vegetative cycles that have suffered in the retainment from lack of completion. Containment, on the other hand, accepts the grievous loss after the deep pain has led to loudly expressed crying and sobbing and the blessed relief of tears. The grief in containment flowed through the person. After a time the healing begins.

The expressed grief has loosened the thoracic diaphragm to which the pelvic diaphragm has responded. The contractions of grief in the upper part of the body have been loosened. The muscles of the head and neck that have helped to keep a brave face for all to see, have gradually relaxed, and there is eventually, in time, a free flow of blood circulating again.

The mask of Parkinson's disorder may be the chronic brave face as it faces the pain of loss. The energetic body will always move towards homeostasis and the inner stasis of the organism will always be under the influence of the energetic movement attempting to reach the organismic periphery. There can be impedance in the body's attempt at expansion.

The tremor could be part of the organism's movement to shake out the tissues susceptible to the influence of the chemostasis resulting from the retention of grief. One patient, recently diagnosed as having the Parkinson's disorder was encouraged to maximise the tremor whenever possible – in social situations such as handing tea to visitors. She learned to treat her difficulty with a light-hearted attitude.

The tremor, which shook the cup on the saucer, was reduced with intention to a degree but she was always nervous that it would be an embarrassment. She found that her change of attitude gave her more confidence on social occasions. When alone she was encouraged to maximise the tremor and shake it out vigorously.

138

The whole organism of the patient suffering from this disorder is vulnerable to many negative changes and the severity of the grief in the patients mentioned would be reflected in developing symptoms. In his book, *Vibrational Medicine*, Dr Richard Gerber[7] reports work done on the study of Parkinson's disorder at the Bob Hope Parkinson Research Centre in America.[8]

Using the Motoyama's AMI electro-puncture diagnostic system the researchers discovered energetic imbalances in the intestinal meridians of many Parkinsonian patients. Dr Gerber goes on to say that:

> It is possible that the common imbalances in the nervous system and digestive system in Parkinson patients are due to an abnormal link between the bowel and the brain.
> The link may be indirect, in that the disease may be dependant on exposure to a third factor that operates upon the pre-existing physiological weaknesses. Abnormalities in the normal functions of absorption and excretion by the intestines may result in a build-up of certain toxic elements in the nervous system.[9]

Biodynamic Psychology, with its concepts of stasis in the gut (the id canal) as a result of undischarged startle patterns and bio-chemical changes in the tissues of the lining and the smooth musculature of the gut, would understand and agree with these findings.

Recently, I was told of some research, which has located production of dopamine in the first part of the duodenum. I am currently awaiting references for this work. The Parkinson Research Centre was, in this instance, conducting research directed at Alzheimer's disease and the possible link with high aluminium levels in those patients who had died from the disease.

Ann's therapeutic progress

It was difficult to get Ann to be committed to attend for her therapeutic journey over the following weeks. Her husband, now very friendly to-

7   Gerber, Richard, *Vibrational Medicine*, Chapter 11, (p. 452), Bear and Co., Santa Fe, New Mexico, 1988.
8   Dr Gerber refers to work carried out at the Bob Hope Parkinson's Research Centre. U.S.A.
9   Gerber, Richard, *Vibrational Medicine*, Bear & Co., Santa Fe, New Mexico, 1988.

wards me, drove her over but said he had little influence on the regularity of her treatments. I had indicated that six treatment sessions would give her a chance to see if any beneficial changes were happening.

I was prepared to see her whenever she decided to attend. She showed very little inner incentive to try anything. Her immobilising depression was entrenched. During the second treatment session, however, she said she loved reading and talked at length of her reading preferences. She demonstrated her keen intellect and her enjoyment when she used her critical faculties.

Ann hated the slow business of undressing and getting on to the massage table. There had to be a compromise. She sat upright in a chair; I was able to treat the rigid muscles of her upper back and neck while at the same time listening for any release sounds from Ann's abdomen. I had to depend on my ears alone because there was difficulty in anchoring the head of the stethoscope. Ann talked freely of what she could and could not do in her daily life. Perhaps she found it easier to talk easily when her back was towards me.

The next session was difficult to arrange. Ann found it difficult to raise the energy to think it through and I was not going to help her with this. Eventually, she decided to attend for the third session in two weeks time. When Ann arrived for the third treatment there was very little change in her condition. The treatment of her neck and shoulders was repeated as she sat upright in a chair.

The biodynamic massage applied was deep Energy Distribution. The musculature appeared to be softer but this could be my optimistic feeling about the need for this technique. Ann talked easily about what she was reading and about her love of clothes and fashion. After I had been treating her neck and shoulders for some minutes, Ann said she would like to try getting on to the massage table again. Some of her outer clothing was already removed. Ann still needed to be raised with three pillows under her shoulders. The stethoscope was anchored over her lower abdomen and I began energy distribution massage over her scalp and face as she lay in the supine position.

The psycho-peristaltic sounds were a mixture of dry electric sounds and at intervals loud watery sounds. They seemed to be more available than previously, but although I paid attention to them I was more anxious to get as much muscle mobilisation as possible in the time that we had.

The pattern of the massage was similar to the treatment of the two previous treatments. However, I needed to give Ann some easy but important homework.

This involved paying attention to the right arm from shoulder to fingertips. After I had completed the energy distribution massage to the whole of her right arm, Ann was asked to feel her arm as I supported it with my two hands. My left hand supported her right elbow and my right hand supported her right hand very lightly. I asked Ann to imagine that her next breath travelled down her right arm down to her fingertips and as she did this I opened her hand and spread her fingers. Ann did this a few times. I asked her to lay her right hand palm down on the massage table and I released her arm from my supporting hands.

With her eyes closed I asked her to pay attention to the stiffness in the fingers of the right hand and to imagine a breath going down her arm as far as her finger tips and a little beyond. Ann did this for a few more breaths and then I took her right hand and stretched it between both of my hands for a few more of Ann's breaths. I asked Ann if she would do this breathing exercise as often as she could particularly when she was watching television – just the right hand initially, until I saw her again.

Respiratory expansion of the thorax and particularly the diaphragm was limited. I used the pulsatory touch technique down the sternum and there were loud mixed sounds from the stethoscope accompanied by a few tentative release breaths. Time dictated what Ann was prepared to use and I completed the treatment by a firm massage to her feet and long distributive strokes to her legs from the pelvis to her feet. A fourth treatment session was arranged for two weeks hence and I wanted to spend more time on her back and leg muscles.

At the end of the first year we had treated the whole of her body with biodynamic techniques but always treating her head, neck and shoulders first as she sat in a chair. In the year Ann had had eighteen hours of treatment which was often piece-meal and with much compromise. Only half of this time was spent in physical therapy the rest was spent in pleasant chat, which we both enjoyed.

At no time in the first year was any psychotherapy attempted. It had been necessary from the outset that Ann should choose to find her own therapeutic tempo and pace. Any deviation from this would have given her a reason not to make the next appointment. Progress in the first year was slow but real. Her depressive feelings were lessening. She enjoyed her reading more as a contribution to life rather than an escape from misery. She was still not prepared to attend more often.

The dryness of the skin of her feet had lessened. There were areas of smoothness without cracks and thickening. She no longer had the feeling of dizziness when she got up from the treatment and this was happening at home when she realised that she could get up in the morning without having to move slowly and let the dizziness subside. The treatment with Energy Distribution massage and mobilisation of the tissues was followed more often by feelings of relaxation and sometimes Ann slept a little after the treatment.

There was a gap at the end of the year when Ann found it impossible for one reason or another to attend for therapy. This lasted for six weeks. Progress in the lessening of her symptoms progressed minimally and there was no recurrence of the dizziness after the treatments or at home. She said that her depressive feelings were not so paralysing though they had not gone away entirely. There was improvement in the rigidity in her fingers and thickening was less. Ann could also extend her fingers and palmar tissues at will and although she forgot to do her exercises from time to time she reported this with humour.

At the end of a year's treatment her facial mask had more mobility and when she smiled her whole face responded. Her stance was still exaggerated in its uprightness, but the shuffling gait had lessened and she was walking with more confidence. Ann bought expensive new shoes. Most encouraging was the improvement in her mood. The muscles of the upper part of her body were becoming softer. Inevitably this resulted in freer flow of blood circulation to the brain tissues. This was needed for the area of the mid-brain where dopamine was produced though there was no real way that any increased production could be measured.

During the second year of treatment, Ann was content to continue the three-weekly treatments. Halfway through the year I received a letter from Ann briefly explaining that she had enclosed a poem she had written after the death of their son. It was poignant and sweet. She asked that I should read it and return it and not talk about it when we met again.

A short time after this she agreed to join her husband on a trip abroad. She had vehemently refused to go anywhere for two years and this she confessed was because her family and friends were unaware of the diagnosis of her condition and, they might guess that she had Parkinson's.

There was another gap in the therapy continuum of six weeks and when Ann returned for more treatment her signs of improvement were more established. She had an impressive tan. She told me at this time that she had resumed her bridge afternoons, 'now that I can deal the cards without making a mess of it'. She was playing every week.

Towards the end of the second year of our relationship Ann began to change her dietary habits. She began a supervised weight loss programme with a well-known organisation. She reduced her weight over a period of six months by two pounds every week. When she had lost forty-two pounds she began to experience severe pain down her left leg as far as the knee.

At this time the neurologist had told her that he no longer needed to see her to check her progress and referred her back to her family doctor for her drug supervision. This pain in her left leg was not new but the other events in her life had taken precedence for her attention. She telephoned for an earlier appointment to discuss the pain. Her family doctor had diagnosed the pain as sciatic and related to the hip replacement. He suggested that Ann should see the orthopaedic consultant for an injection into the leg. Ann thought that her body was adjusting to the weight loss and that the pain was as a result of the adjustment. She preferred that she and I attended to this together.

This was the best evidence so far that Ann was in charge once more and she decided to have weekly treatments for a while. The treatment involved Ann lying prone on the massage table as her preferred position. She was able to lie comfortably like this without anything more than a small pillow under her head.

The tissues of the entire leg were mobilised down to bone level; particular attention was paid to the distribution of the sciatic nerve pathway. There was no pain in any of the tissues of the limb. The psychoperistalsis sounds were most responsive to the mobilisation down the outer aspects of the gluteals and down the semi tendinosus. The sounds lessened as the lower limb was massaged.

Further mobilising massage was applied to the whole of the spine and the right leg. Ann turned over on to her left side and was, on this occasion, content to rest for a few moments. When she rose from the table she experienced a pain free limb. Ann asked for two or three weekly sessions to be on the safe side. The pain did not return.

Ann was pleased that her diagnosis had been the correct one. Ann has had forty-seven treatments of the biodynamic body techniques and little psychotherapy. She has reached the stage where, after two and a half years, she feels she can trust her body to tell her when things are in need of attention and she will ask for it. Her newly acquired look gives her much pleasure. She feels less worried about depressive feelings that surface occasionally.

The latest occurred when she woke up the morning after she had had the treatment for the sciatic pain. Ann said

> I know that something more than the pain went away, perhaps it was what caused the depression.

She then said

> I sometimes feel so good that I realise I have forgotten to take my pills. When I very occasionally wake up in the morning feeling depressed, I think of something to do and do a chore. I get up and do it and then realise that I am no longer depressed. I am no longer worried about winter, which was always a misery for me.

A very prolonged therapeutic programme was probably good for Ann in the long run. It took time for her to develop her feedback system; most of her insights were spontaneous. Ann's decision to reduce her weight came from her and was never suggested by me.

Summary

Biodynamic concepts and treatment can have a positive and prolonged effect on Parkinson's syndrome as observed in the cases I have treated. It is very necessary that the therapist understand as much as possible of the neuro-physiology as is known currently. In this way attention to the person will result in as clear an intention as is possible. The intention will be to distribute the life energy through the blood circulation by energy distribution massage.

Emotionally static areas will inhibit the healthy free-flow of the blood supply. In all the patients treated the biodynamic principles and techniques were the same throughout. All patients were treated on a weekly session basis. Ann was the exception. There is no way of knowing if her progress would have been different had she had weekly treatments. I doubt whether she would have deviated from the way she behaved.

There is also no way that the therapist can know when a layer of old and buried emotion may surface. It is always wise to tell the patient that whatever surfaces in the two or three days following a treatment is part of the undoing of the old patterns. Sometimes these days are palatable sometimes even joyful. Sometimes there can be a heaviness in the body or poor rhythms of sleep If the patient is prepared then they are patient with themselves. Often the patient expresses gratitude for having been warned.

Glossary of Terms Used in Biodynamic Psychology and Psychotherapy

Abreaction
The psychoanalytic term for the removal, by revival and expression, of the emotion associated with the forgotten ideas of the event, which first produce the emotion.

Amygdala
A structure deep within the brain. One of the pleasure centres of the brain.

Armouring
The physical and/or emotional defences shown by an individual. The armour serves to keep potentially explosive emotions bottled up within the organism and to ward off the emotions of others.

Biofield
The electromagnetic field surrounding living organisms.

Bioenergetics
A modification by Alexander Lowen of Wilhelm Reich's Vegetotherapy. Lowen practised this modification of the Reichian techniques.

Biorelease
A discipline developed by Mona Lisa Boyesen. Its aim is to increase spontaneous emotional discharge, to encourage self-regulation and increase knowledge of the nature of body/mind synthesis.

Centre
The supreme centre from the ancient Chinese culture is the place of the soul, the upper field of elixir. It is the physical centre of gravity in the human body. The ancient Japanese called it the Hara.

Chemostatic Fluid
This fluid can be understood in the light of Gerda Boyesen's important concepts of neurosis. It is the physiological component underlying Freud's psychological concept of residual effect.

Chiropractic
An assortment of manipulative techniques applied to the spinal column in order to assist the body healing.

Cosmic Laws
Wilhelm Reich conceived and developed these cosmic insights and described them as Laws 1 and 2. Gerda Boyesen describes the phenomena in the *Collected Papers of Biodynamic Psychology*.

Cosmic Superimposition
This is the transformation of the cosmic energy into electricity and ultimately bioelectricity in the animate form.

Deep-Draining
A massage technique developed by Gerda Boyesen from training she had received from the Norwegian physiotherapist, Aadal Bulow Hansen. It was first known as psycho-motoric massage.

DNA.
Deoxyribonucleic Acid. A macro molecule which encodes the genetic information.

Effleurage
A physiotherapeutic massage of long flowing strokes to the body directed towards the heart.

Ego and Id
The psychoanalytic terms for the conscious and unconscious. According to biodynamic philosophy the id is the canal for the movement of instinctive drives. In 1923 Freud wrote that the 'ego appears as that part of the id which has been modified by the direct influence of the external world'.

148

Emptying
A biodynamic touch technique where the touch is held until a psycho-peristaltic response occurs.

Energy
The primordial energy that permeates the cosmos according to Wilhelm Reich. It is behind all processes in nature.

Energy Blockage
An interruption of the natural flow of life energy due to disruption at a chakra level.

Energy Distribution
The name given to an energy massage technique developed by Ebba Boyesen. Energy Distribution is a biodynamic massage intended to be non-provocative. It is used to heighten a person's capacity for feelings of well being.

Energy Field
The life energy requires a field in order to flow.

Enzyme
A protein with the specialised action of catalysing a chemical reaction in the body and giving it direction.

Fast Up-going Petrissage
A massage technique developed for a biodynamic therapeutic treatment. Useful in the treatment of entrenched depressive states.

Gentle Mirror Breathing
Ebba Boyesen – (also *Mirror Breathing*) – A very gentle breathing technique, biodynamically developed. This technique appears to calm the breathing tract and reduce the harmful tensions in the muscles of the upper thorax and the throat area. The person lifts his or her chin and breathes very gently as though breathing on to a mirror. This is a very calming self-help technique that can be used when under stress. I have used it when a male patient, with a previous history of coronary disease,

became very agitated when experiencing chest pains whilst he was waiting for the doctor and ambulance. I encouraged him to use this technique and he found it helpful.

The Great Mimicker
A term used by some chiropractic practitioners. It describes the impact on the human organism affecting the ileo-caecal valve area. A disturbance of the ileo-caecal valve junction in mild pathology can be spoken of as open or closed. Symptoms may be mistaken as having other origins, hence the term.

Hara
In the Japanese language it means the belly but particularly describes the place deep within the body, below the navel. It is the body's centre of gravity.

Homeostasis
A term used to describe the condition and balance following a healthy ability to deal with the stresses of life. The body systems obtain harmony.

Hyperaemia
An excessive accumulation of blood in a particular part of the body.

Hypertensive and Hypotensive
Descriptive words for tissue in the organs that have responded to disturbances in the energy of the organism. The terms in general refer to a lack of emotional expression in the individual.

The Id Canal
The biodynamic concept of the gut as the conduit for the instinctive drives. A Gerda Boyesen concept.

Id energy
Emotional energetic charge that can move up and down the id canal as it seeks discharge. For example, it can drift upwards towards the throat and larynx where it can find verbal or sound expression.

Idiopathic
Describes a disease not occasioned by, or caused by, another disease.

Ileo-caecal valve
A valve between the ileum section of the small intestine and the ascending colon.

Libido
The biodynamic interpretation is that the pleasurable flow of cosmic energy through the body is not confined to the psychoanalytic interpretation of sexual energy.

Life Energy
Described by Wilhelm Reich as orgone energy. It is the cosmic energy that permeates the cosmos. It fills all space and is the agency for movement. Life energy penetrates all matter and responds to the cosmic laws as described by Reich. In ancient civilisations it was known as, for instance *chi, ki* or *prana*.

Lifting
A biodynamic technique used in biodynamic massage therapy to loosen the major joints in tune with the patient's breathing rhythm.

Mask
The mask can be observed in a patient's depressive state. It is protective of the emotional state locked into the underlying tissues. The tissues have responded with immobility that can contain chemostatic tissue fluid. Greek and Roman actors in the ancient world wore the human figure of the head.

Myelin Sheath
A fatty tissue that develops along axons in some parts of the central nervous system. If it is damaged, the individual may eventually suffer from the disease of Multiple Sclerosis.

Neuron (e)
A nerve cell.

Neurotransmitter
A chemical or protein released at the synaptic membrane designed to continue the passage of messages from one nerve to the adjacent nerve.

Orgonomy
Doctor Elsworth Baker, following the influence of Wilhelm Reich, gave his name to techniques in Orgonomy. It is also the name given to a Bio-release massage developed by Mona Lisa Boyesen. Reich built a centre for the study of the Orgone and Orgonomy and named it *Orgonon*.

Orgonomy Massage
Orgonomy massage acts to stimulate the plasma currents of the deeper musculature.

Palpation
This is a touch that aims to judge the condition of tissues and organs below the surface of the body.

Petrissage
A massage technique used to stimulate muscle tissue. In biodynamic psychology the fast upgoing massage technique is a fast, firm variety of this technique. It can be used in entrenched states of a depressive illness by changing the stasis of the blood supply so that the patient feels a difference in their body totality.

Plasma-Faradic/Plasma-Galvanic principle
A Gerda Boyesen concept for the action of life-energy as it passes through life tissue. The Plasma-Faradic has a cleansing function. The Plasma-Galvanic has a toning function.

Peristalsis
An action that is wave-like in its contractions in successive circles. It is found in the alimentary tract. These movements serve to propel the contents of the tract along its length.

Prone
The action of lying face down.

Psycho-Orgastic
A term used in a dance exercise as taught by Ebba Boyesen. Its origins are primitive and in many cultures. The term implies that there is a reservoir of sexual energy stored in the sacral area. This energy is released in normal health, as the organism requires it. It can, however, be locked into that area due to emotional malfunction. This biodynamic technique can help to reverse the malfunction. The force of energy in that area is also known to yogic devotees as the snake, the kundalini energy.

Psychosomatic
A term used to convey the acceptance that the body and mind are linked in the development of some body disorders.

Psychogenic
A term used to convey the understanding that an illness may be the result of a psychological disorder.

Pulsation
A movement of the life energy in a living organism from the centre to the periphery. A point of stillness is then followed by a movement of the life energy from the periphery to the centre.

Psycho-Peristalsis
The term given to Gerda Boyesen's insight when she noted that the alimentary tract has a secondary function. This function acts as a digester of stress products, and works in parallel with the digestion of nutrients in the alimentary tract.

Segmental Theory
Reich conceived that the current of orgone (life) energy flowed vertically along the body axes. He also saw that the neurotic, muscular armour rings were segmented at right angles to the vertical axes, for instance, an emotional disturbance in the eye muscles he saw as an ocular ring – the ocular segment.

Startle Reflex Pattern
The autonomic nervous system response to danger to the organism.

Stasis
A stoppage in the flow of the body fluids. An important aspect of biodynamic psychology is that emotional stasis can develop into stasis on the bio-chemical level – chemostasis. Homeostasis is when the organism is balanced in all its functions.

Streamings
Vegetative streamings are experienced after the dissolution of spasms and tensions in the body. They may feel like tingling sensations rippling under the skin.

Stretching
Can be experienced as a reflex that the body muscles need to elongate in order to contract down to the feeling of relief. The stretch reflex can be experienced on an even deeper level when the life energy has pierced and has flowed through tissue that had been immobilised.

Super Ego
Freud's concept of a psychological function that controls the function of the ego – the individual's conscience. Freud developed a structural account of the mind in which the uncoordinated instinctual drives were called the id, the organised realistic part, the ego and the critical moralising function, the super ego.

Supine
The attitude of lying face up.

Synchronicity
A term which means relating to, or exhibiting, the concurrence of events in time. A phenomenon of importance in Carl Jung's philosophy.

Tapôtement
A massage technique involving percussion of the body by the practitioner. The sides of the hands are used in rapid alternation over particular muscle groups.

T. Cells
For instance T. helper cells travel by way of the blood and stimulate B cells to manufacture anti-bodies.

Tonus
A healthy condition of the body tissues. An increase in tonus, or tone, can disturb the balanced functioning of tissues. A decrease in tonus can similarly disturb the balance. The biodynamic therapist would pursue the reasons for the imbalance and take appropriate therapeutic action.

Tryptophan
An enzyme of complex metabolism which starts the conversion of amino acids to neurotransmitters. It requires B6 and Magnesium to do this. B6 is involved in tryptophan conversion to seratonin.

Vegetative Release
The phenomenon in biodynamic therapy where an unresolved part of the startle reflex pattern achieves completion with a subsequent, harmonious autonomic nervous system.

Vegetotherapy
A therapy developed by Wilhelm Reich. He found a muscular counterpart to his character armour concept and through the vegetative (autonomic) nervous system, developed techniques to dissolve the armour.

Vermiform Appendix
A residual, small organ attached to the caecum and the lower portion of the colon.

Visceral Armour
An important concept conceived by Gerda Boyesen when she formulated her hypothesis of the alimentary tract as a conduit for the Id energy and an organ for the digestive processes applied to residual stress hormones.

Bibliography and suggested reading

Bentov, Itzhak, *Stalking the Wild Pendulum,* Destiny Books, 1977.

Best, Simon, and Smith, Cyril W., *Electromagnetic Man*, J.M. Dent and Sons Ltd., 1990.

Boadella, David, *Embryology and Therapy*, Abbotsbury Publications, 1979.

Boadella, David, *Wilhelm Reich – The Evolution of his Work*, Arkana Edition, Routledge and Kegan Paul, 1985.

Boyesen, Gerda, and Boyesen, Mona Lisa, *Collected Papers of Biodynamic Psychology*, Volumes 1 and 2, Biodynamic Psychology Publications, London, Reprinted from *Energy and Character*, Abbotsbury Publications, 1969-79.

Boyesen, Gerda, 'Oscar the Case History of a Manic Depressive', *Collected Papers of Biodynamic Psychology,* Biodynamic Psychology Publications London, reprinted from *Energy and Character,* Volume 6, No.1, Abbotsbury Publications, 1975.

Boyesen, Mona Lisa, 'The Infant and the Alpha', *Journal of Biodynamic Psychology* No 2, Biodynamic Psychology Publications, London, 1981.

Bozler, E., 'Action Potentials and the Conduction of Excitation in Muscle', *Biological Symposia* 3, 95-109, University of Oslo, 1941. (Translated from the Norwegian by Bente Schmid).

Brennan, Barbara Ann, *Hands of Light,* Bantam Books, 1988.

Brennan, Barbara Ann, *Light Emerging,* Bantam Books, 1989.

Capra, Fritjof, *Tao of Physics,* Flamingo 3rd Edition, 1982.

Carmichael, Stephen W., and Winkler, Hans, 'Chromaffin Cells', *Scientific American*, August, 1985.

Cherniss, Cary, *Beyond Burnout*, Rutgers University, Routledge, London, 1999.

Chilton-Pearce, Joseph, *The Magical Child*, Bantam Books, 1978.

Coghill, Roger, *Electro Healing in The Medicine of the Future*, Thorsons, London, 1991.

Davidson, John, *The Web of Life,* C.W. Daniel Co. Ltd., Saffron Walden, 1988.

Dossey, Larry, *Space, Time and Medicine,* Shambala Publications Inc., Boulder, Colorado, USA, Routledge & Kegan Paul, London, 1982.

Evans, John, *Mind, Body and Electromagnetism*, Element Books, 1989.

Ferguson, Marilyn, *The Aquarian Conspiracy*, Paladin, 1982.

Freud, Sigmund, 'The Ego and the Id – Anatomy of the Mental Personality', *New Introductory Lectures in PsychoAnalysis*, 1932.

Gauquelin, Michael, *How Cosmic Atmosphere Energies Influence Your Health,* Aurora Printing, 1984.

Gerber, Richard, M.D., *Vibrational Medicine*, Bear and Co., Santa Fe, New Mexico, 1988.

Green, J.H. *Basic Clinical Physiology*, Oxford University Press, London, 1982.

Groddeck, Georg, *The Book of the It,* NMD Publications Co., 1928.

Journal of Biodynamic Psychology, Numbers 1, 2 and 3, Biodynamic Psychology Publications, London, 1981, 1982, 1983.

Koestler, Arthur, *Janus – A Summing-Up*, Pan Books, 1979.

Kreiger, Dolores, *Therapeutic Touch*, Englewood Cliffs, NJ, Prentice Hall, 1979.

Le Gros Clark, W.E., *Tissues of the Body*, Oxford University Press, 1975.

Montagu, Ashley, *Touching – The Human Significance of the Skin*, Harper and Row Publisher Inc., New York, 1989.

Nunneley, Peg, *The Biodynamic Philosophy and Treatment of Psychosomatic Conditions,* Volume Two, Peter Lang, 2000.

Odent, Michel, *Primal Health*, Century Hutchinson Ltd., 1986.

Oldfield, Harry, Coghill, Roger, *The Dark Side of The Brain*, Element Books,1988.

Pierrakos, John, M.D., *Core Energetics*, Life Rhythm Publications, 1987.

Reich, Wilhelm, *The Discovery of the Orgone*, Volume 2 'The Cancer Biopathy', Orgone Institute Press, 1948.

Reich, Wilhelm, 'Cosmic Orgone Energy and Ether' *Orgone Energy Bulletin*, Volume 1, No. 4, 1949.

Rowan, J. and Dryden, W., *Innovative Therapies in Britain*, Open University Press, 1988.

Sanella, Lee, M.D., *The Kundalini Experience – Psychosis or Transcendence*, Integral Publishing, 1987.

Saxon Burr, Harold, *Blueprint for Immortality*, C.W. Daniels Co. Ltd., 1983.

Schiff, Michael, *The Memory of Water*, Thorsons, 1995.

Scott, Mary, *Kundalini in the Physical World*, Arkana, London, 1987.

Selye, Hans, *The Stress of Life,* Mc Graw-Hill Book Company, 1978.

Setekleiv, Johannes, 'The Spontaneous Rhythm Activity in Smooth Musculature', *Tidskrift Norske Laegerforen,* University of Oslo. 1964. (Translated from the Norwegian by Bente Schmid).

Sills, Franklyn, *The Polarity Process*, Element Books Ltd., 1989.

Spencer, Herbert, *Principles of Biology,* London, 1872.

St John, Robert, *Metamorphosis and the Metamorphic Technique.* To be published by the Metamorphic Association, London.

Stone, Randolph, M.D. *Complete Collected Works of Dr Randolph Stone,* CRCS Publications, USA and Canada, 1986.

Weber, Renee, *The Holographic Paradigm*, Shambala,1982.

Wendell-Smith, C.P., and Williams, P.L., *Basic Human Embryology*, Pitman Publishing, London, 1994.

Biodynamic Psychology and Psychotherapy

edited by Mary Molloy
Institute of Biodynamic Psychology and Psychotherapy

Biodynamic Psychology and Psychotherapy is a dynamic biological and psychological approach to the theory of mind and human development. It was founded by Mrs Gerda Boyesen, the Norwegian Clinical Psychologist and Reichian Analyst over forty years ago. Its distinctive approach is derived from the psychoanalytical concepts of Freud and Jung and especially Wilhelm Reich. Its methodology is also based upon concepts and practices developed by psychodynamic, humanistic, cognitive, transpersonal, neo-reichian, integrative and other human potential approaches. It considers that the psyche's true potential arises from the alignment of the body, mind, soul and spirit. The profound establishment of spontaneous life movements in the body and mind, and the cognitive, conscious experience of the life energy in each person remains a key focus for all biodynamic theory and practice.

The series Biodynamic Psychology and Psychotherapy will present core texts, selected writings and descriptive accounts of academic, clinical and personal experiences related to the biodynamic field. It will include a presentation of the many new, creative, innovative and exciting applications of the biodynamic approach in a variety of settings. Treatment for specific diseases, psychosomatic conditions and psychopathologies will be outlined and discussed from the biodynamic perspective, and the potential for a new understanding of body, mind, spirit and emotion will be introduced. The series will also include specific training manuals, textbooks and research derived from clinical practice in the field.